Clinical Management of Male Infertility

Giorgio Cavallini • Giovanni Beretta
Editors

Clinical Management
of Male Infertility

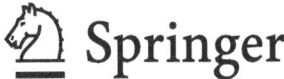
Springer

Editors
Giorgio Cavallini
Andrological Unit
Gynepro Medical Team
Bologna
Italy

Giovanni Beretta
Andrological and Reproductive
Medicine Unit
Centro Demetra
Firenze
Italy

ISBN 978-3-319-08502-9   ISBN 978-3-319-08503-6 (eBook)
DOI 10.1007/978-3-319-08503-6
Springer Cham Heidelberg New York Dordrecht London

Library of Congress Control Number: 2014952787

© Springer International Publishing Switzerland 2015
This work is subject to copyright. All rights are reserved by the Publisher, whether the whole or part of the material is concerned, specifically the rights of translation, reprinting, reuse of illustrations, recitation, broadcasting, reproduction on microfilms or in any other physical way, and transmission or information storage and retrieval, electronic adaptation, computer software, or by similar or dissimilar methodology now known or hereafter developed. Exempted from this legal reservation are brief excerpts in connection with reviews or scholarly analysis or material supplied specifically for the purpose of being entered and executed on a computer system, for exclusive use by the purchaser of the work. Duplication of this publication or parts thereof is permitted only under the provisions of the Copyright Law of the Publisher's location, in its current version, and permission for use must always be obtained from Springer. Permissions for use may be obtained through RightsLink at the Copyright Clearance Center. Violations are liable to prosecution under the respective Copyright Law.
The use of general descriptive names, registered names, trademarks, service marks, etc. in this publication does not imply, even in the absence of a specific statement, that such names are exempt from the relevant protective laws and regulations and therefore free for general use.
While the advice and information in this book are believed to be true and accurate at the date of publication, neither the authors nor the editors nor the publisher can accept any legal responsibility for any errors or omissions that may be made. The publisher makes no warranty, express or implied, with respect to the material contained herein.

Printed on acid-free paper

Springer is part of Springer Science+Business Media (www.springer.com)

Contents

1. **Introduction** 1
   Paolo Turchi, Giovanni Beretta, and Giorgio Cavallini

2. **Prevalence, Definition, and Classification of Infertility** 5
   Paolo Turchi

3. **Interpretation of Sperm Analysis** 13
   Giovanni Beretta

4. **Diagnosis of Infertility** 23
   Edoardo S. Pescatori

5. **General Therapeutic Approach to Male Infertility** 33
   Giorgio Cavallini

6. **Azoospermia** 41
   Giorgio Franco, Leonardo Misuraca, and Gabriele Tuderti

7. **Varicocele and Infertility** 55
   Giovanni Beretta

8. **Chromosomic Causes of Infertility** 63
   Gianni Paulis

9. **Male Idiopathic (Oligo) ± (Astheno) ± (Terato)-Spermia** 79
   Giorgio Cavallini

10. **Obesity and Male Infertility** 89
    Carlo Maretti

11. **Unexplained Couple Infertility (Male Role)** 99
    Giorgio Cavallini

12. **Inflammatory Infertility** 105
    Giorgio Cavallini and Gianni Paulis

13. **Testicular Pathology** 119
    Fulvio Colombo, Giorgio Gentile, and Alessandro Franceschelli

14	**Endocrine Infertility**	135
	Giorgio D. Piubello	
15	**Iatrogenic Infertility**	145
	Giovanni Beretta	
16	**Dietary Complements and Phytotherapy**	153
	Bruno Giammusso	
17	**Environmental Pollution and Infertility**	165
	Giorgio Cavallini	
18	**The Role of the Andrologist in Assisted Reproduction**	173
	Giorgio Cavallini and Giovanni Beretta	
19	**Sexual Problems and Infertility**	179
	Giovanni Beretta	
Index		185

Introduction

Paolo Turchi, Giovanni Beretta, and Giorgio Cavallini

The clinical management of couple infertility suffers from a way of thinking still widely diffused today among those working in the field, who often consider the understanding of the male factor of infertility too vague and its remedies not yet supported by solid scientific evidence. Consequently it often happens that couples are initiated directly to assisted reproduction techniques (ART), even in the presence of a male factor, undiagnosed or untreated [1, 2]. Unilateral handling of reproductive care, according to this common way of thinking, should provide the couple with the best chances of procreation. In fact, there are four strong reasons to favor bilateral management of the infertile couple, including an assessment of the male.

Firstly, infertility should be considered a disease. It can be an expression of sometimes serious disorders not yet diagnosed at the time of the search for pregnancy [3, 4]. A comprehensive male infertility evaluation may allow to detect significant disease(s) that otherwise would have remained undiagnosed if the evaluation of the male factor were limited to seminal examination only. Recent studies have suggested that male infertility may be associated with reduced longevity [5] and that male factor infertility is an increased risk factor for certain malignancies [6, 7]. Furthermore, the condition of an infertile male can cause psychological and marital stress [8–10]. Quantifying this risk, it has been estimated that for every 15 couples evaluated, in 1 couple (6 %) the male partner has a significant medical condition [11].

P. Turchi, MD (✉)
Andrology Unit, Azienda USL 4 di Prato, Prato, Italy
e-mail: paolo.turchi@fastwebnet.it, pturchi@usl4.toscana.it

G. Beretta
Andrological and Reproductive Medicine Unit, Centro Demetra,
via Della Fortezza 6, Firenze 50129, Italy
e-mail: giovanniberetta@libero.it

G. Cavallini
Andrological Unit, Gynepro Medical Team, Bologna, Italy
e-mail: giorgiocavallini@libero.it

These figures highlight the concept that not to provide infertile males with an appropriate diagnostic evaluation should be regarded as an error and/or omission by the physician and a missed opportunity, objectively difficult to justify.

Secondly, a correct andrologic diagnostic workout may unveil infertility factors in about 70 % of infertile males [12]. Many of such factors are correctable or treatable, with the perspective ideally to allow the couple to spontaneously conceive, but also to have better chances of success when exposed to ART [13–16].

Thirdly, scientific evidence suggests that considering the high cost, success rates, and possible side effects of ART, early efforts to improve male fertility appear to be an attainable and worthwhile primary goal. The main results obtained concern evidence-supported indications regarding other causes of male infertility, and their early detection and treatment [17].

Lastly, it should be appreciated that the modern andrologist is no longer a specialist acting according to personal experience and common sense only. Scientific evidence and ensuing clinical guidelines are in fact today available. The skills of the andrologist today encompass internal medicine, endocrinology, seminology, microbiology, molecular biology surgery, and genetics. Pertinent scientific societies, according to the available peer reviewed literature, have produced guidelines, recommendations and diagnostic/therapeutic algorythms. Such advances in the andrologic field allow today infertile males to be properly evaluated and potentially treated, making the andrologist the male infertility specialist that is equipped with the latest medical knowledge.

References

1. Nicopoullos JD, Gilling-Smith C, Ramsay JW (2004) Male-factor infertility: do we really need urologists? A gynaecological view. BJU Int 93:1188–1190
2. Tournaye H (2006) Evidence-based management of male subfertility. Curr Opin Obstet Gynecol 18:253–259
3. Honig SC, Lipshultz LI, Jarow J (1994) Significant medical pathology uncovered by a comprehensive male infertility evaluation. Fertil Steril 62:1028–1034
4. Salonia A, Matloob R, Gallina A, Abdollah F, Saccà A, Briganti A, Suardi N, Colombo R, Rocchini L, Guazzoni G, Rigatti P, Montorsi F (2009) Are infertile men less healthy than fertile men? Results of a prospective case–control survey. Eur Urol 56(6):1025–1031
5. Jensen TK, Jacobsen R, Christensen K, Nielsen NC, Bostofte E (2009) Good semen quality and life expectancy: a cohort study of 43,277 men. Am J Epidemiol 170(5):559–565
6. Walsh TJ, Schembri M, Turek PJ, Chan JM, Carroll PR, Smith JF, Eisenberg ML, Van Den Eeden SK, Croughan MS (2010) Increased risk of high-grade prostate cancer among infertile men. Cancer 116(9):2140–2147
7. Walsh TJ, Croughan MS, Schembri M, Chan JM, Turek PJ (2009) Increased risk of testicular germ cell cancer among infertile men. Arch Intern Med 169(4):351–356
8. Smith JF, Walsh TJ, Shindel AW, Turek PJ, Wing H, Pasch L, Katz PP, Infertility Outcomes Program Project Group (2009) Sexual, marital, and social impact of a man's perceived infertility diagnosis. J Sex Med 6(9):2505–2515
9. Eisenberg ML, Smith JF, Millstein SG, Walsh TJ, Breyer BN, Katz PP, Infertility Outcomes Program Project Group (2010) Perceived negative consequences of donor gametes from male and female members of infertile couples. Fertil Steril 94(3):921–926

10. Nelson CJ, Shindel AW, Naughton CK, Ohebshalom M, Mulhall JP (2008) Prevalence and predictors of sexual problems, relationship stress, and depression in female partners of infertile couples. J Sex Med 5(8):1907–1914
11. Kolettis PN, Sabanegh ES (2001) Significant medical pathology discovered during a male infertility evaluation. J Urol 166:178–180
12. Jungwirth A, Giwercman A, Tournaye H, Diemer T, Kopa Z, Dohle G, Krausz C, European Association of Urology Working Group on Male Infertility (2012) European Association of Urology guidelines on male infertility: the 2012 update. Eur Urol 62(2):324–332
13. Esteves SC, Oliveira FV, Bertolla RP (2010) Clinical outcome of intracytoplasmic sperm injection in infertile men with treated and untreated clinical varicocele. J Urol 184(4):1442–1446
14. Cocuzza M, Cocuzza MA, Bragais FM, Agarwal A (2008) The role of varicocele repair in the new era of assisted reproductive technology. Clinics (Sao Paulo) 63(3):395–404
15. Showell MG, Brown J, Yazdani A, Stankiewicz MT, Hart RJ. (2011). Antioxidants for male subfertility. Cochrane Database Syst Rev (1):CD007411
16. Valenti D, La Vignera S, Condorelli RA, Rago R, Barone N, Vicari E, Calogero AE (2013) Follicle-stimulating hormone treatment in normogonadotropic infertile men. Nat Rev Urol 10(1):55–62
17. Campagne DM (2013) Can male fertility be improved prior to assisted reproduction through the control of uncommonly considered factors? Int J Fertil Steril 6(4):214–223

Prevalence, Definition, and Classification of Infertility

2

Paolo Turchi

2.1 Definition

Infertility is defined by the World Health Organization (WHO) as "a disease of the reproductive system defined by the failure to achieve a clinical pregnancy after 12 months or more of regular unprotected sexual intercourse" [1]. Infertility can also be defined on the basis of demographic considerations, such as "an inability of those of reproductive age (15–49 years) to become or remain pregnant within 5 years of exposure to pregnancy" [2] or as "an inability to become pregnant with a live birth, within 5 years of exposure based upon a consistent union status, lack of contraceptive use, non-lactating and maintaining a desire for a child" [3]. The WHO also defines infertility from an epidemiologic perspective: "women of reproductive age (15–49 years) at risk of becoming pregnant (not pregnant, sexually active, not using contraception and not lactating) who report trying unsuccessfully for a pregnancy for 2 years or more." No definition considers male infertility as a specific condition, and in only one, contained in the 5th edition of the WHO *Laboratory Manual for the Examination and Treatment of Human Sperm*, has the male factor been cited: "Infertility is the inability of a sexually active, non-contracepting couple to achieve pregnancy in 1 year. The male partner can be evaluated for infertility or subfertility using a variety of clinical interventions, and also from a laboratory evaluation of semen" [4]. In this statement, reference is made to the need for a comprehensive evaluation of the infertile male.

Once considered a disorder of inconvenience, infertility has been classified as a disease in the US regulatory Americans with Disabilities Act [5]. Indeed, infertility in women was ranked the fifth highest serious global disability (among rural populations younger than 60 years) [6]. This change of view also applies to men. A disease is any deviation from or interruption of the normal structure or function of any

---

P. Turchi
Andrology Unit, Azienda USL 4 di Prato, Prato, Italy
e-mail: paolo.turchi@fastwebnet.it, pturchi@usl4.toscana.it

part, organ, system, or combination thereof of the body that is manifested by a characteristic set of symptoms or signs. Based on this definition, male infertility meets these criteria [7] and thus should accordingly, be considered a disease.

2.2 Epidemiology

While most studies agree that infertility affects approximately 15–20 % of all couples [8–11], data relating to male infertility are more uncertain. An epidemiologic study of male infertility in fact presents a clinical problem because fertility is a couple-related concept and male fecundity (i.e., his biological capacity to reproduce) is a component of the fertility rate. Both male and female partners make an independent contribution to a couple's fertility, but the outcomes of fertility are only fixed in terms of pregnancy rate or births. It is often difficult to determine which partner makes the greatest contribution to a couple's disease, and this difficulty is a feature of infertility, in which there are no pathognomonic findings to confirm a diagnostic certainty. This difficulty is also an important limitation of epidemiologic studies, in which the male factor is often undervalued and underestimated.

Epidemiologic studies of male infertility are also severely limited by several other factors. First, traditionally the couple's infertility is addressed by evaluating the woman while male diagnostics is often confined to a semen analysis. Semen quality and quantity are the most widely used biological markers of male fertility and are a source of essential information in assessing the fertility of a couple, but they correlate with indices of subfertility, such as time to pregnancy (TTP), in addition to sexual activity and several other conditions [12]. Semen analysis is poorly predictive of the male fertility status, mainly giving information about the status of the male genital tract and, thus, only indirect indications of potential male fertility. Moreover, semen analysis is an operator-dependent examination and has a high coefficient of variability [13]. Classification of the male condition of fertility/infertility based on the seminal characteristics is an influential factor that limits the understanding of the problem. Furthermore, male infertility is not a specific disease subject to documentation as is, for example, a prostate cancer, which is easily detectable within large-scale databases. In addition, it is usually evaluated and treated in the private outpatient setting, and clinical data are not stored in the public health system databases. Therefore, quantifying the actual burden of the male component is often impossible. The consequence is a lack of data with which to track diagnoses and treatments of a disease, and difficulty in quantifying its causes and frequency. Another factor limiting the understanding of the epidemiologic problem, and which contributes to the loss of data related to male infertility, is the frequent use of empiric treatments of male factor infertility, such as the in vitro fertilization (IVF) that primarily treats the female partner. In general, IVF programs require that an exact cause is assigned for the woman, whereas the male factor is classified only as present or not present. When a male cause is reported, it is almost always based only on seminal data without undertaking a clinical assessment, making data partial and generic [14, 15].

2.3 Incidence

The majority of studies examining the incidence and prevalence[1] of male infertility have been conducted in specific geographic regions. In these studies, the incidence of male factor infertility varied considerably depending on the region considered. For example, a study conducted in Siberia reported female and male factors to account for 52.7 % and 6.4 %, respectively [10], whereas a Nigerian study revealed a high prevalence of male infertility [16]. In this study, male factor infertility was estimated at 42.4 % whereas female factors were estimated at 25.8 %. In 20.7 % of couples, both partners were affected. Sexual promiscuity and sexually transmitted diseases (and inadequate treatment) have been implicated in the high rate of male factors [16]. Epidemiologic studies are numerous but, even considering all the data available today, none is able to define the incidence of male infertility. Male factor infertility can vary widely based on geography (e.g., Siberia vs Nigeria) and inherent risk factors. Evaluating existing literature, a component of male factor infertility may range widely, from 6 to 50 %, with many groups estimating 30–50 % [17–20]. Perhaps the only consistent aspect found in the scientific literature is that male infertility is variable with a multitude of contributory factors (race, country, geography, socioeconomic variables, environmental and occupational exposures, the fertility of the partner, and so forth), many of which require further research to be better characterized. To understand the approximation of these data it should be re-emphasized, however, that the true extent of male infertility is probably underestimated because of the frequent lack of assessment of the male in the diagnostic workup of infertile couples. Eisenberg et al. [21] have evaluated the frequency of evaluation of male infertility using data from the National Survey of Family Growth, and have found that 18–27 % of men in infertile couples were not evaluated. Overall, these data suggest that male factor infertility is a significant component of global infertility and needs better quantification, using population-based studies conducted on a large scale, to help physicians fill these gaps in understanding.

2.4 Classification

The nosology of male infertility, despite the growing attention it receives from medical research, is still difficult to define. On the one hand a growing burden of the male component of the infertile couple is described, with studies reporting a decline in male fertility over the years [22–25]. On the other hand, except for some specific causes of infertility such as cryptorchidism and genetic causes, other infertility factors, such as varicocele or genitourinary tract infections, often remain hypothetical and are not investigated. Male infertility therefore continues to be classified as being due to poor semen quality (oligozoospermia, asthenozoospermia, or teratozoospermia alone or in

---

[1] Incidence is defined as the number of new cases of a disease in a specific population at risk over a specific period of time. Prevalence is defined as the total number of cases of disease (both old and new) present in a specified population at a single point in time.

combination) of unknown causes, which does not contribute to increased knowledge about the etiology [26]. A correct clinical evaluation of the infertile male would, instead, identify an infertility factor in 60–70 % of cases (Table 2.1). In 30–40 % of cases, no cause of male infertility can be found; these men, affected by oligoasthenoteratozoospermia syndrome, might be defined as having idiopathic male infertility.

Table 2.1 Male infertility causes and associated factors, and percentage of distribution in 10,469 patients

Diagnosis	Unselected patients ($n=12,945$)	Azoospermic patients ($n=1,446$)
All	100 %	11.2 %
Infertility of known (possible) cause	42.6	42.6
Maldescended testes	8.4	17.2
Varicocele	14.8	10.9
Sperm autoantibodies	3.9	–
Testicular tumor	1.2	2.8
Others	5.0	1.2
Idiopathic infertility	30.0	13.3
Hypogonadism	10.1	16.4
Klinefelter syndrome (47, XXY)	2.6	13.7
XX male	0.1	0.6
Primary hypogonadism of unknown cause	2.3	0.8
Secondary (hypogonadotropic) hypogonadism	1.6	1.9
Kallmann syndrome	0.3	0.5
Idiopathic hypogonadotropic hypogonadism	0.4	0.4
Residual after pituitary surgery	<0.1	0.3
Others	0.8	0.8
Late-onset hypogonadism	2.2	–
Constitutional delay of puberty	1.4	–
General/systemic disease	2.2	0.5
Cryopreservation due to malignant disease	7.8	12.5
Testicular tumor	5.0	4.3
Lymphoma	1.5	4.6
Leukemia	0.7	2.2
Sarcoma	0.6	0.9
Disturbance of erection/ejaculation	2.4	–
Obstruction	2.2	10.3
Vasectomy	0.9	5.3
Cystic fibrosis (congenital bilateral absence of vas deferens)	0.5	3.1
Others	0.8	1.9

From Jungwirth et al. [27] and Thonneau et al. [26]

Table 2.2 Classification and distribution of the causes of male infertility

Pretesticular	5–10 %
Testicular	65–75 %
Post-testicular	10–20 %

Table 2.3 Main factors associated with male infertility

Cryptorchidism
Genetic causes
Varicocele
Testicular tumors
Testicular trauma
Genitourinary tract infections (testis, epididymis, prostate, seminal vesicles)
Iatrogenic causes (surgery, chemotherapy, radiotherapy)
Systemic diseases
Twisting of the spermatic cord

Table 2.4 Main risk factors associated with male infertility

Age	
Lifestyle	
	Cigarette smoke
	Substances abuse (alcohol, cannabis derivatives, opioids)
	Sedentary lifestyle/obesity
	Scrotal temperature (clothing, underwear, occupational exposure to heat, regular sauna)
	Exposure factors and/or toxic environmental/occupational
	Family history of infertility and/or recurrent poliabortivity

When we consider male factor infertility, we imply a series of possible causal factors divided into pretesticular causes (inadequate stimulation of the testis by gonadotropin), testicular causes (diseases of the testis), and post-testicular causes (seminal tract obstructions, ejaculatory disorders, erectile dysfunction) (Table 2.2). As almost none of the causes can be considered a definitive factor of infertility, it is preferable to define each condition as a male infertility associated factor whenever a clinical evaluation of the infertile male is performed Table 2.3). In addition, many risk factors are associated with a worsening of semen quality (Table 2.4), which is attracting great attention and should be considered in the process of collecting the medical history, but for which, at present, the scientific evidence is not sufficiently strong.

References

1. Zegers-Hochschild F, Adamson GD, de Mouzon J, Ishihara O, Mansour R, Nygren K, Sullivan E, Vanderpoel S (2009) International Committee for Monitoring Assisted Reproductive Technology (ICMART) and the World Health Organization (WHO) revised glossary of ART terminology. Fertil Steril 92(5):1520–1524

2. Rutstein SO, Iqbal HS (2004) Infecundity, infertility, and childlessness in developing countries. Demographic and health surveys (DHS) comparative reports No. 9. ORC Macro and World Health Organization Geneva, Switzerland, Calverton
3. Mascarenhas MN, Flaxman SR, Boerma T, Vanderpoel S, Stevens GA (2012) National, regional, and global trends in infertility: a systematic analysis of 277 health surveys. PLoS Med 9(12):e1001356
4. World Health Organization (2010) WHO laboratory manual for the examination and processing of human semen, 5th edn. World Health Organization, Geneva
5. Meacham RB, Joyce GF, Wise M, Kparker A, Niederberger C (2007) Male infertility. J Urol 177(6):2058–2066
6. Krahn GL (2011) World Report on Disability: a review. World Health Organisation and World Bank. Disabil Health J 4(3):141–142
7. Winters BR, Walsh TJ (2014) The epidemiology of male infertility. Urol Clin North Am 41:195–204
8. Sharlip ID, Jarow JP, Belker AM, Lipshultz LI, Sigman M, Thomas AJ, Schlegel PN, Howards SS, Nehra A, Damewood MD, Overstreet JW, Sadovsky R (2002) Best practice policies for male infertility. Fertil Steril 77(5):873–882
9. Gunnell DJ, Ewings P (1994) Infertility prevalence, needs assessment and purchasing. J Public Health Med 16(1):29–35
10. Philippov OS, Radionchenko AA, Bolotova VP, Voronovskaya NI, Potemkina TV (1998) Estimation of the prevalence and causes of infertility in Western Siberia. Bull World Health Organ 76(2):183–187
11. Sabanegh E, Agarwal A (2011) Male infertility. In: Wein A (ed) Campbell-Walsh urology, 10th edn. Elsevier Saunders, Philadelphia, pp 616–647
12. Olsen J, Ramlau-Hansen CH (2014) Epidemiologic methods for investigating male fecundity. Asian J Androl 16:17–22
13. Filimberti E, Degli Innocenti S, Borsotti M, Quercioli M, Piomboni P, Natali I, Fino GM, Cagliaresi C, Criscuoli L, Gandini L, Biggeri A, Maggi M, Baldi E (2013) High variability in results of semen analysis in andrology laboratories in Tuscany (Italy): the experience of an external quality control (EQC) programme. Andrology 1(3):401–407
14. Smith JF, Walsh TJ, Shindel AW, Turek PJ, Wing H, Pasch L, Katz PP (2009) Sexual, marital, and social impact of a man's perceived infertility diagnosis. J Sex Med 6(9):2505–2515
15. Jensen TK, Jacobsen R, Christensen K, Jacobsen R, Christensen K, Nielsen NC, Bostofte E (2009) Good semen quality and life expectancy: a cohort study of 43,277 men. Am J Epidemiol 170(5):559–565
16. Ikechebelu JI, Adinma JI, Orie EF, Ikegwuonu SO (2003) High prevalence of male infertility in southeastern Nigeria. J Obstet Gynaecol 23(6):657–659
17. Mosher WD, Pratt WF (1991) Fecundity and infertility in the United States: incidence and trends. Fertil Steril 56(2):192–193
18. Brugh VM 3rd, Matschke HM, Lipshultz LI (2003) Male factor infertility. Endocrinol Metab Clin North Am 32(3):689–707
19. Leke RJ, Oduma JA, Bassol-Mayagoitia S, Bacha AM, Grigor KM (1993) Regional and geographical variations in infertility: effects of environmental, cultural, and socio economic factors. Environ Health Perspect 101(Suppl 2):73–80
20. Tielemans E, Burdorf A, te Velde E, Weber R, van Kooij R, Heederik D (2002) Sources of bias in studies among infertility clients. Am J Epidemiol 156(1):86–92
21. Eisenberg ML, Lathi RB, Baker VL, Westphal LM, Milki AA, Nangia AK (2013) Frequency of the male infertility evaluation: data from the national survey of family growth. J Urol 189(3):1030–1034
22. Skakkebaek NE, Jorgensen N, Main KM, Toppari J (2006) Is human fecundity declining? Int J Androl 29(1):2–11, 3,11,12
23. Auger J, Kunstmann JM, Czyglik F, Jouannet P (1995) Decline in semen quality among fertile men in Paris during the past 20 years. N Engl J Med 332(5):281

24. Carlsen E, Giwercman A, Keiding N, Skakkebaek NE (1992) Evidence for decreasing quality of semen during past 50 years. BMJ 305(6854):609–613
25. Menchini-Fabris F, Rossi P, Palego P, Simi S, Turchi P (1996) Declining sperm counts in Italy during the past 20 years. Andrologia 28(6):304
26. Thonneau P, Marchand S, Tallec A, Ferial ML, Ducot B, Lansac J, Lopes P, Tabaste JM, Spira A (1991) Incidence and main causes of infertility in a resident population (1,850,000) of three French regions (1988–1989). Hum Reprod 6(6):811–816
27. Jungwirth A, Giwercman A, Tournaye H, Diemer T, Kopa Z, Dohle G, Krausz C, European Association of Urology Working Group on Male Infertility (2012) European Association of Urology guidelines on male infertility: the 2012 update. Eur Urol 62(2):324–332

Interpretation of Sperm Analysis

Giovanni Beretta

3.1 Is Sperm Analysis an Indicator of Male Infertility?

Sperm analysis is an important fertility test for infertile couples, and it is suggested that this test be performed before any treatments even if a female problem has been resolved. It is unacceptable to subject a woman to medical procedures and tests without knowing the status of her partner's semen. Semen analysis has long represented the standard test for evaluating male fertility and remains a cornerstone; however, it is a poor predictor of fertility [1].

The World Health Organization (WHO) guidelines on sperm analysis are based on percentiles, which in turn are based on a group of men who fathered children in a time window of 1 year or less. The lower acceptable numbers represent the fifth percentile of this group. In other words, fewer than 5 % of the men who fathered a child in the past year had semen parameter measurements below these cutoffs. This implies that having better or worse numbers does not necessarily mean that a man will or will not be able to father a child. The semen parameters are merely guidelines to consider when investigating the potential causes of infertility.

Diagnosis is important in the management of male infertility, but "infertility" in itself is not a diagnosis but a symptom, like pain. Sperm analysis is only the first step; all male patients with abnormal sperm should have a full clinical history taken and should undergo a complete clinical examination.

G. Beretta
Andrological and Reproductive Medicine Unit, Centro Demetra,
via Della Fortezza 6, Firenze 50129, Italy
e-mail: giovanniberetta@libero.it

In general, a man is asked to abstain from any ejaculations for 3 to 5 days before the test. In the laboratory it is important to use a cup, provided by the lab, because some materials are toxic to spermatozoa; if the sperm is obtained at home the sample should be brought to the laboratory within approximately 1 h.

The sperm analysis must include the evaluation of both macroscopic and microscopic parameters; if found to be abnormal, the test should be performed on multiple ejaculates before characterizing a man as infertile [2].

The biological variation of seminal parameters further diminishes the clinical significance of the most recent WHO reference values.

Data indicate that there are variations in semen parameters between men in different geographic regions and even between samples from the same individual [3, 4].

3.2 Macroscopic Parameters

Semen is made up of more than just sperm; in fact, less than 5 % of semen consists of sperm. Healthy semen includes fluid from the testes, the seminal vesicles, the prostate gland, and the bulbourethral glands.

Normal ejaculate is between 1.5 and 6 mL of fluid. Absence of seminal fluid after orgasm (*aspermia*) occurs in males with diabetic neuropathy, following surgical procedures, or after the intake of sympatholytic drugs. In some of these cases, because the nervous plexus is damaged, there may be retrograde ejaculation into the bladder, and an examination of the postejaculatory urine should be conducted.

Volume <1.5 mL (*hypospermia*) may be due to the loss of a portion of the ejaculate during collection, incomplete orgasm, or incorrect abstinence. pH <7.0 may indicate absence of seminal vesicles or obstruction/subobstruction of the ejaculatory ducts. If pH is >8.0, this may indicate hypogonadism with accessory gland impairment, inflammation, or intake of narcotics.

Appearance and *semen color* seem to be insignificant in assessing sperm fertilization potential.

A translucent aspect can denote the absence of spermatozoa, whereas an opaque sample may indicate the absence of sperm cellular components. Red color may indicate an excessive number of erythrocytes (*hematospermia*) and yellow color the presence of jaundice.

When semen is ejaculated it is thick and gelatinous, to help it adhere to the cervix. The semen eventually liquefies within 20–30 min of ejaculation. *Absence of coagulation* denotes possible obstruction or agenesia of seminal vesicles with secondary lack of secretions. *Delayed liquefaction* may indicate a problem with the prostate, the seminal vesicles, or the bulbourethral glands, also known as the male accessory glands.

Viscosity is another parameter that is considered abnormal if the length of a thread exceeds 50 mm; in these cases there is low sperm motility and the sperm transportation can be compromised.

3 Interpretation of Sperm Analysis

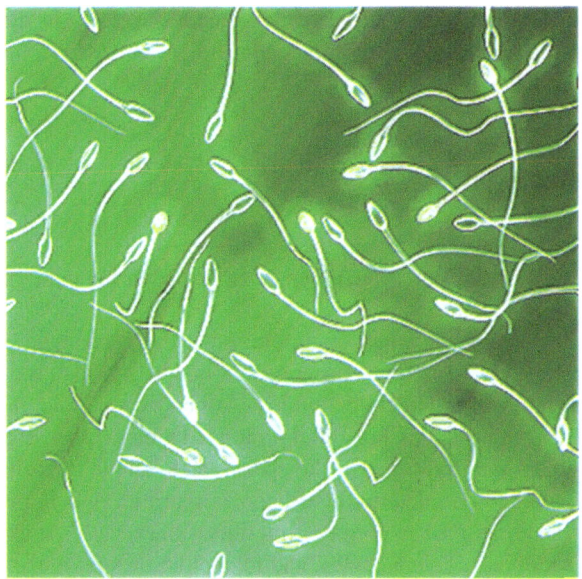

3.3 Microscopic Parameters

3.3.1 Sperm Concentration

Sperm count is in millions per milliliter of semen. Normal samples have more than 15 million spermatozoa per milliliter.

The cutoff of 15 million spermatozoa/mL has been suggested in 2010 by the WHO as the lower normal value for sperm concentration in an ejaculate. Normal semen has more than 39 million in the whole ejaculate [5].

In a study evaluating two semen specimens from each of the male partners in 765 infertile couples and 696 fertile couples, subfertile men had sperm concentrations of $<13.5 \times 10^6$/mL [6].

Another study that evaluated 166 male factor infertility patients and 56 proven fertile donors has suggested the concentration of 31.2×10^6/mL as a prognostic factor for fertility status [7].

On the other hand, the literature describes significant overlap in threshold sperm concentration between fertile and infertile men.

Oligozoospermia, a low sperm concentration, is indicated when sperm concentration falls below $5-10 \times 10^6$/mL, and may be due to the loss of a portion of the ejaculate, partial obstruction of the genital tract, drugs, or genetic abnormalities. Other factors include the use of various medications, such as aspirin or nitrofurantoin, and excessive heat exposure.

Azoospermia, the absence of spermatozoa, may be caused by complete obstruction of sperm transport, hypogonadism, and iatrogenic causes (chemotherapy), or idiopathic factors that are most probably genetic in origin. In these cases, the semen analysis must be repeated with cytocentrifugation of the sample to confirm the azoospermia [8].

3.3.2 Sperm Motility

Spermatozoa are graded according to their ability to swim.

Sperm that swim in a progressive manner are graded as having rapid or sluggish motility.

Sperm motility is considered as compromised if the percentage of progressive motility falls below 32 % and total (progressive + nonprogressive) motility is below 40 % within 60 min of sample collection [5]. Asthenozoospermia, the presence of low sperm motility, can occur as a result of prolonged time to processing of collected samples. Containers may be toxic to the sperm, and sample exposure to extreme temperature or sunlight can determine asthenozoospermia. A long period of abstinence can also be a cause of poor sperm motility. Other causes include axonemal deformities of spermatozoa, leukocytes, and idiopathic factors. Asthenozoospermia is also most commonly seen with antisperm antibodies. The observation of sperm clumping combined with low sperm motility is a further indication of the presence of antisperm antibodies [9].

The presence of severe asthenozoospermia necessitates an investigation of sperm viability and identification of necrozoospermia (nonviable spermatozoa).

A *vitality test* is suggested when the number of immotile sperm is >60 %. This is a staining technique that identifies whether the immotile sperm are dead or just immotile, and is reported as percentage vitality. The normal value is 58 % or above.

3.3.3 Sperm Morphology

The shape and size of the sperm are assessed on a stained preparation. The 2010 WHO guidelines encourage the use of Kruger's strict criteria, based on the research of Kruger and Menkeveld [10].

In men whose partners are able to conceive within 12 months, a lower normal value of 4.0 % has been suggested for morphologically normal spermatozoa [5].

Debate is still ongoing regarding the morphologic criteria that should be used and which one offers the most predictive power for in vivo and in vitro fertility.

In advocating the use of the strict criteria, the WHO suggests >4 % as a cutoff point for correlation with positive in vitro fertilization (IVF) outcomes [11].

It is important to note that other studies have found the strict criteria to be of less value in predicting IVF outcomes [12].

3.3.4 Non-Sperm Cellular Components

Immature germ cells are present in oligozoospermia, where the ejaculates usually have low sperm counts.

3 Interpretation of Sperm Analysis

Table 3.1 Distribution of values for semen parameters from men whose partners became pregnant within 12 months of discontinuing contraceptive use [5]

Parameter (units)	N	Centile								
		2.5	5	10	25	50	75	90	95	97.5
Semen volume (mL)	1,941	1.2	1.5	2.0	2.7	3.7	4.8	6.0	6.8	7.6
Sperm concentration (10^6 per mL)	1,859	9	15	22	41	73	116	169	213	259
Total sperm number (10^6 per ejaculate)	1,859	23	39	69	142	255	422	647	802	928
Progressive motility (PR, %)	1,780	28	32	39	47	55	62	69	72	75
Non-progressive motility (NP, %)	1,778	1	1	2	3	5	9	15	18	22
Immotile spermatozoa (IM, %)	1,863	19	22	25	31	39	46	54	59	65
Normal forms (%)	1,851	3	4	5.5	9	15	24.5	36	44	48
Vitality (%)	428	53	58	64	72	79	84	88	91	92

Special attention should be given to the concentration of leukocytes in the seminal ejaculate. Leukocytes are normally present in the seminal fluid, but a concentration above 1×10^6/mL is considered abnormal [5]. A higher than normal white blood cell (WBC) count is known as leukocytospermia, which may indicate infection. However, some men may have leukocytospermia without any active infection or male fertility impairment. In fact, anywhere from 5 to 20 % of men tested may be found to have leukocytospermia. A positive correlation has been observed between leukocyte count and the total count of microorganisms in semen samples. An optimal sensitivity/specificity ratio appears at 0.2×10^6 WBC/mL semen [13] (Table 3.1).

The excessive presence of leukocytes may be detrimental to spermatozoa, owing to their excessive production of reactive oxygen species (ROS) and cytotoxic cytokines [14].

The presence of erythrocytes is not always indicative of reproductive tract abnormality, while the presence of microorganisms is an indication of genital tract infection [15].

3.4 Sperm Function Tests

Semen analysis is mainly used to estimate male fertility potential, but clinical research has shown that normal semen analysis might not reflect defects in sperm function. Sperm function testing is used to determine if the sperm have the capacity to reach and fertilize oocytes. A variety of tests is available to evaluate different aspects of these functions [16, 17].

Our knowledge of the molecular mechanisms regulating sperm function continues to grow, as do the opportunities for new diagnostic tests; for example, recent studies emphasize the importance of nuclear DNA integrity and compaction [18–20].

3.4.1 Test of Sperm Capacitation

Capacitation is a series of structural and biochemical changes that spermatozoa go through to be able to fertilize an oocyte.

All processes take place in the female genital tract, but with capacitation media can be induced in vitro. It is thought to have a role in preventing the release of lytic enzymes until spermatozoa reach the oocyte. One of the signs of capacitation is the display of hyperactivation by spermatozoa. At present, the clinical value of sperm capacitation testing remains to be determined [21].

3.4.2 Testing for Antibody Coating of Spermatozoa

It has been known for more than 100 years that an immune response can be generated against the antigens present on the surface of spermatozoa. The presence of antisperm antibodies can be suggested on the basis of excessive sperm agglutination. Antibodies may block the penetration of cervical mucus by spermatozoa, or prevent sperm binding and penetration of zona pellucida.

Immunologic protection to sperm antigens are provided by the tight junctions of Sertoli cells forming the blood-testis barrier.

The antigenic capacity of semen can be ascribed to the fact that spermatogenesis begins during puberty, when the immune system is able to respond to antigenic stimulations. The spermatozoon evokes an immune response when exposed to the systemic immune defense system under conditions whereby this barrier gets disrupted and leads to the formation of antisperm antibodies, such as testicular torsion, vasectomy, and testicular trauma [9].

Two current methods of detecting antibodies bound to the surface of motile sperm are the Mixed Agglutination Reaction assay (MAR test; only for immunoglobulin G) and the immunobead-binding assay (for immunoglobulins A, G, and M).

A positive finding of >50 % motile sperm with attached beads is considered to be clinically significant [22, 23].

3.4.3 Tests of Sperm DNA Damage

DNA damage is interconnected with poor semen parameters, e.g., low sperm concentration, low motility, and high levels of reactive oxygen species. Fertilization in mammals involves the direct interaction of the sperm and the oocyte, fusion of the cell membranes, and union of male and female gamete genomes. Although a small percentage of spermatozoa from fertile men also possess detectable levels of DNA damage, which is repaired by oocyte cytoplasm, there is evidence to show that the spermatozoa of infertile men possess substantially more DNA damage and that this damage may adversely affect reproductive outcomes [24, 25]. There appears to be a threshold of sperm DNA damage, which can be repaired by oocyte cytoplasm (ie, abnormal chromatin packaging, protamine deficiency), and beyond which embryo development and pregnancy are impaired [26, 27].

3.4.3.1 Direct Tests
(a) Terminal deoxynucleotidyl transferase-mediated deoxyuridine triphosphate nick end-labeling (TUNEL) assay
(b) DNA oxidation measurement

3.4.3.2 Indirect Tests
(a) Sperm chromatin structure assay (SCSA)
(b) Sperm chromatin dispersion assay
(c) Sperm fluorescence in situ hybridization analysis (FISH)

Overall, even if there are some data to suggest that sperm DNA damage is associated with poor pregnancy outcome after standard IVF, there is no significant relationship between sperm DNA damage and fertilization rate or pregnancy outcomes at IVF or IVF/intracytoplasmic sperm injection [5, 28–31].

According to the Practice Committee of the American Society for Reproductive Medicine, significant intraindividual variations exist for the sperm chromatin structure assay, making precise conclusions problematic [32].

3.5 Conclusions

Semen analysis is essential in estimating male fertility, but is not a direct measure of it. Abnormalities in the semen analysis can occur for numerous reasons, such as incomplete collection by the patient. Illness, fever, stress, and various medications can also affect sperm quality.

Confirmation of a true sperm problem requires at least a second test. Each variable alone is not a suitable predictor of the fertility status, and has to be considered in the context of the other parameters and the clinical setting.

References

1. Lewis SE (2007) Is sperm evaluation useful in predicting human fertility? Reproduction 134:31–40
2. Keel BA (2006) Within- and between-subject variation in semen parameters in infertile men and normal semen donors. Fertil Steril 85:128–134
3. Alvarez C, Castilla JA, Martinez L, Ramirez JP, Vergara F, Gaforio JJ (2003) Biological variation of seminal parameters in healthy subjects. Hum Reprod 18:2082–2088
4. Jorgensen N, Andersen AG, Eustache F et al (2001) Regional differences in semen quality in Europe. Hum Reprod 16:1012–1019
5. World Health Organisation (2010) WHO laboratory manual for the examination and processing of human semen, 5th edn. WHO, Geneva
6. Guzick DS, Overstreet JW, Factor-Litvak P et al (2001) Sperm morphology, motility, and concentration in fertile and infertile men. N Engl J Med 345:1388–1393

7. Nallella KP, Sharma RK, Aziz N, Agarwal A (2006) Significance of sperm characteristics in the evaluation of male infertility. Fertil Steril 85:629–634
8. Jarow JP, Espeland MA, Lipshultz LI (1989) Evaluation of the azoospermic patient. J Urol 142:62–65
9. Beretta G, Chelo E, Marzotto M, Zanollo A (1993) Anti-sperm antibodies in dyspermia in spinal cord injury patients. Arch Ital Urol Androl 65(2):189–192
10. Kruger TF, Acosta AA, Simmons KF et al (1987) New method of evaluating sperm morphology with predictive value for human in vitro fertilization. Urology 30:248–251
11. Coetzee K, Kruge TF, Lombard CJ (1998) Predictive value of normal sperm morphology: a structured literature review. Hum Reprod Update 4:73–82
12. Morgentaler A, Fung MY, Harris DH, Powers RD, Alper MM (1995) Sperm morphology and in vitro fertilization outcome: a direct comparison of World Health Organization and strict criteria methodologies. Fertil Steril 64:1177–1182
13. Punab M, Loivukene K, Kermes K, Mandar R (2003) The limit of leucocytospermia from the microbiological viewpoint. Andrologia 35:271–278
14. Pasqualotto FF, Sundaram A, Sharma RK, Borges E Jr, Pasqualotto EB, Agarwal A (2008) Semen quality and oxidative stress scores in fertile and infertile patients with varicocele. Fertil Steril 89:602–607
15. Agarwal A, Bragais FM, Sabanegh E (2008) Assessing sperm function. Urol Clin North Am 35:157–171, vii
16. Ombelet W, Bosmans E, Janssen M, Cox A, Vlasselaer J, Gyselaers W et al (1997) Semen parameters in a fertile versus subfertile population: a need for change in interpretation of semen testing. Hum Reprod 12:987–993
17. Sigman M, Baazeem A, Zini A (2009) Semen analysis and sperm function assays: what do they mean? Semin Reprod Med 27:115–123
18. Sakkas D et al (1998) Sperm nuclear DNA damage and altered chromatin structure: effect on fertilization and embryo development. Hum Reprod 13(Suppl 4):11–19
19. Aitken RJ, Krausz CG (2001) Oxidative stress, DNA damage and the Y chromosome. Reproduction 122:497–506
20. Virro MR et al (2004) Sperm chromatin structure assay (SCSA) parameters are related to fertilization, blastocyst development, and ongoing pregnancy in in vitro fertilization and intracytoplasmic sperm injection cycles. Fertil Steril 81:1289–1295
21. Tesarik J (1989) Appropriate timing of the acrosome reaction is a major requirement for the fertilizing spermatozoon. Hum Reprod 4:957–961
22. Mortimer D (1994) Practical laboratory andrology. Antisperm antibodies. Oxford University Press, Oxford, pp 111–125
23. Jarow JP, Sanzone JJ (1992) Risk factors for male partner antisperm antibodies. J Urol 148:1805–1807
24. Evenson DP, Jost LK, Marshall D, Zinaman MJ, Clegg E, Purvis K et al (1999) Utility of the sperm chromatin structure assay as a diagnostic and prognostic tool in the human fertility clinic. Hum Reprod 14:1039–1049
25. Zini A, Bielecki R, Phang D, Zenzes MT (2001) Correlations between two markers of sperm DNA integrity, DNA denaturation and DNA fragmentation, in fertile and infertile men. Fertil Steril 75:674–677
26. Ahmadi A, Ng SC (1999) Fertilizing ability of DNA-damaged spermatozoa. J Exp Zool 284:696–704
27. Cho C, Jung-Ha H, Willis WD, Goulding EH, Stein P, Xu Z et al (2003) Protamine 2 deficiency leads to sperm DNA damage and embryo death in mice. Biol Reprod 69:211–217
28. Bungum M, Humaidan P, Axmon A, Spano M, Bungum L, Erenpreiss J et al (2007) Sperm DNA integrity assessment in prediction of assisted reproduction technology outcome. Hum Reprod 22:174–179
29. Benchaib M, Lornage J, Mazoyer C, Lejeune H, Salle B, François Guerin J (2007) Sperm deoxyribonucleic acid fragmentation as a prognostic indicator of assisted reproductive technology outcome. Fertil Steril 87:93–100

30. Lin MH, Kuo-Kuang Lee R, Li SH, Lu CH, Sun FJ, Hwu YM (2008) Sperm chromatin structure assay parameters are not related to fertilization rates, embryo quality, and pregnancy rates in *in vitro* fertilization and intracytoplasmic sperm injection, but might be related to spontaneous abortion rates. Fertil Steril 90:352–359
31. Frydman N, Prisant N, Hesters L, Frydman R, Tachdjian G, Cohen-Bacrie P et al (2008) Adequate ovarian follicular status does not prevent the decrease in pregnancy rates associated with high sperm DNA fragmentation. Fertil Steril 89:92–97
32. The Practice Committee of the American Society for Reproductive Medicine (2013) The clinical utility of sperm DNA integrity testing. Fertil Steril 99:673–677

Diagnosis of Infertility

Edoardo S. Pescatori

Whenever a couple has not conceived after 1 year of unprotected intercourse, both partners should undergo a thorough medical examination. An earlier evaluation is suggested in the presence of a known male (i.e., history of cryptorchidism) or female (i.e., age over 35 years) infertility risk factor or if a man wishes to know his fertility potential [1].

The justification for male evaluation by an andrologist relies on the fact that a male factor is solely responsible in about 20 % of infertile couples and is contributory in another 30–40 % [2, 3]. It is presently recommended that, to categorize infertility, both partners should be investigated simultaneously [4]. The goals of a male evaluation for infertility are to identify causes of infertility that after correction could allow natural conception, to identify causes of infertility that after correction could increase the chances of success of assisted reproduction technologies (ARTs), and to explore underlying conditions that, in additionto being related to infertility, could pose a risk for the man's health.

4.1 Andrologic Evaluation for Male Infertility: The Initial Office Visit

The minimum andrologic evaluation for male infertility should include a complete medical history, physical examination, and the evaluation of at least two semen analyses [1]. The physical evaluation is usually complemented by the ultrasonographic evaluation of the scrotal content and, if indicated, the prostate. All of these tests can be carried out during a single andrologic office visit. Additional

---

E.S. Pescatori, MD
Andrology Service, Hesperia Hospital, Via Arquà 80/A, Modena 41125, Italy
e-mail: edopes@alice.it

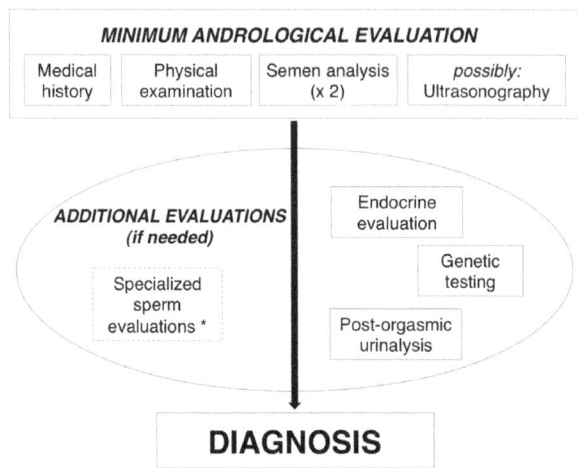

Fig. 4.1 Andrologic workup flow chart: *specialized sperm evaluations are presently considered experimental (WHO)

investigations may be appropriate, should specific problems emerge at the initial office visit. These tests chiefly comprise endocrine evaluation, genetic testing, post-orgasmic urinalysis, and specialized sperm evaluations (Fig. 4.1). The components of the andrologic office visit are detailed here.

4.1.1 Medical History

The medical history should investigate all possible causes that may affect the fertility potential of the man. The following areas should be addressed.

4.1.1.1 Reproductive History
Did the man under investigation formerly induce pregnancy or pregnancies with the present or other partners? If so, this would suggest that medical attention be focused more on the present female partner. Should a history of spontaneous abortions be present, this should direct one's attention to sperm DNA evaluations.

4.1.1.2 Occupational History
Professions at risk of affecting fertility, such as direct and prolonged exposure to high temperatures (e.g., kitchen work) and exposure to gonadotoxic agents (e.g., pesticides), should be noted. According to the specific agent, fertility may improve after 1–2 spermatogenetic cycles (3–6 months) after discontinuation of exposure.

4.1.1.3 Lifestyle Risk Factors
Smoke [5–7], excessive alcohol [8] and coffee [9] intake, recreational drugs [10], elevated body mass index (BMI) [11, 12], and low physical activity [13] also have been linked to impaired male fertility; modifying such risk factors may have a positive impact on male fertility.

Fig. 4.2 Prader orchidometer

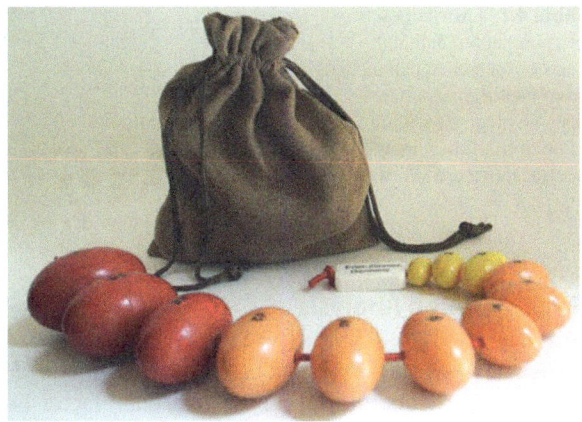

4.1.1.4 Andrologic History
The possible occurrence of the following conditions should be investigated: undescended testis and age of orchiopexy, testis torsion and outcome, former inguinoscrotal surgery such as for inguinal hernia repair, former prostate surgery, pubertal/prepubertal mumps-related orchitis, pubertal development, anosmia, former neoplasia and related treatments, current and recent medications, current and recent genitourinary symptoms or infections, and recent episodes of high fever.

4.1.1.5 Sexual History
The patient should be asked about libido, quality of erection, intercourse frequency, ejaculation, and possible sexual distress related to reproductive difficulties or timed sex.

4.1.2 Physical Examination

In the man evaluated for infertility, physical examination is more informative by far than in the woman: male genitalia are external and easily evaluated, even without the aid of ultrasonography. Moreover, the main male sexual accessory gland, the prostate, can be digitally palpated through the anus.

The andrologic physical evaluation should comprise: evaluation of secondary sexual characteristics, presence of (pseudo-)gynecomastia, penis inspection with attention to location of the external urethral meatus, and digital rectal examination of the prostate.

A detailed evaluation of the scrotal content is of paramount importance. Testes should be assessed for bilateral presence, location (in place, vs retained, vs ectopic), size (according to Prader orchidometer; Fig. 4.2), consistency, and presence of nodules. Epididymides should be evaluated for their presence, possible dilatations, and associated cysts. Bilateral presence of deferent ducts should be ascertained. The presence of varicocele, and its grading [14], should be sought while in orthostasis (Fig. 4.2).

Table 4.1 Distribution of values at 5th and 50th centiles for semen parameters from men whose partners became pregnant within 12 months of discontinuing contraceptive use (WHO)

Parameter	(Units)	Centile	
		5th	50th
Semen volume	(mL)	1.5	3.7
Sperm concentration	(10^6/mL)	15	73
Total motility (PR + NP)	(%)	40	61
Normal forms	(%)	4	15

PR progressive motility, *NP* nonprogressive motility

4.1.3 Semen Analysis

Semen analysis is the cornerstone of the laboratory evaluation of the infertile male, and helps to define the severity of the male factor [1]. The 2010 World Health Organization (WHO) *Laboratory Manual for the Examination and Processing of Human Semen* details the present standards of semen analysis and the related laboratory protocols [15], and every laboratory performing semen analyses should comply with such standards.

In general, laboratory reports of semen analysis define values within normal as those values that do not fall below the lower reference limit (fifth centile). When critically evaluating sperm analysis reports, it should be remembered that the fifth centile indicates values below which only 5 % of the observations of fertile men will fall, and not the average values of fertile men whose partners had a time to pregnancy of 12 months or less [15]. Table 4.1 lists the latest WHO sperm parameter reference values of the 5th and 50th centiles, with the aim of providing the reader with a more critical interpretation of sperm analysis.

It should always be remembered that semen parameters within the 95 % reference interval do not guarantee fertility; nor do values outside these limits, in isolation from other clinical data, necessarily indicate male infertility or abnormality: a man's semen characteristics need to be interpreted in conjunction with his clinical information [16] (Table 4.2).

4.1.4 Ultrasonography Evaluation of Testes and Prostate

Usually the andrologic physical evaluation of the male is complemented by ultrasonographic evaluation of scrotal content and, if indicated, the prostate.

Testis sonography adds useful information regarding the structure of testicular tissue (Fig. 4.3a: microlithiasis), the possible presence of nonpalpable tumors, accurate definition of testes volumes, details of epididymis, and varicocele definition (using Doppler ultrasonography performed while in orthostasis).

If there are clues of obstructive pathology, a transrectal ultrasonogram may unveil an intraprostatic obstructive cyst (Fig. 4.3b). Obstructive intraprostatic cysts should be suspected in the presence of reduced semen volume or even azoospermia, normal-sized testes with distended epididymis, and ejaculatory discomfort/pain.

4 Diagnosis of Infertility

Table 4.2 Some examples of medical history, physical examination, semen analysis data, and possible underlying pathology

Medical history	Physical examination	Semen analysis	Suspected
Former prostate surgery	–	Reduced/absent sperm at orgasm	Retrograde ejaculation
Anosmia/delayed puberty	Cryptorchidism	–	Kallmann syndrome
Inguinal hernia repair	Distended epididymis	Oligospermia	Deferent ischemic damage
Low libido	Altered sexual characters	OAT	Hypogonadism
Low libido	Small firm testes	Azoospermia	Klinefelter syndrome
Postpubertal parotitis	Small soft testes	Azoospermia/cryptozoospermia	Postviral testicular damage
–	Varicocele	OAT	Causal role of varicocele
Pain at ejaculation	Prostatic tender "nodule"	Low semen volume	Obstructive intraprostatic cyst
–	Small testes	Normal volume, azoospermia	Nonobstructive azoospermia
–	Distended epididymis	Low volume, azoospermia	Obstructive azoospermia
Recent fever	Painful epididymis	Two million WBC/mL OAT	Infection

OAT oligoasthenoteratospermia, *WBC* white blood cells

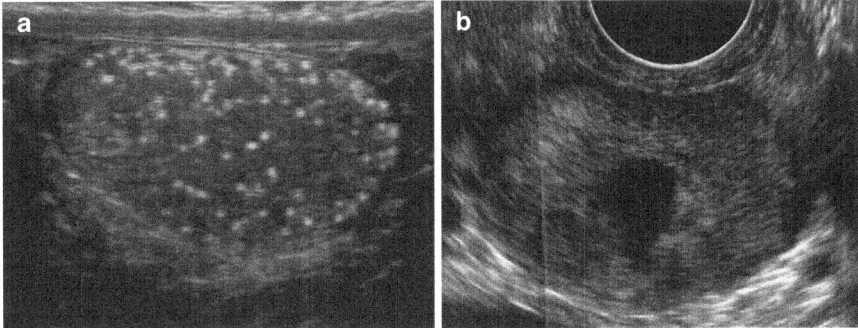

Fig. 4.3 Possible ultrasonographic findings (**a**): testicular microlithiasis; (**b**): intraprostatic obstructive cyst

4.2 Andrologic Evaluation for Male Infertility: Additional Investigations

Some elements gathered during the initial andrologic office visit may prompt further diagnostic workup. The more frequent aspects of additional investigation are endocrine status, genetic testing, postorgasmic urinalysis, and specialized sperm evaluations.

Table 4.3 Simplified endocrinologic differential diagnoses in the presence of altered sperm analysis

FSH	LH	TT	Interpretation
>	>	<	Primary hypogonadism: the problem is the testis
<	<	<	Secondary hypogonadism: the problem is hypothalamus/hypophysis
>	N	N	Possibly: maturation arrest, germinal aplasia, genetic causes
N	N	N	Nonendocrine causes vs functional hypogonadotropic hypogonadism

FSH follicle-stimulating hormone, *LH* luteinizing hormone, *TT* total testosterone, *N* normal

4.2.1 Endocrine Evaluation

It is appropriate to perform an endocrine evaluation whenever medical history and physical findings suggest an endocrinopathy, in the presence of a low sperm count, and if there is concomitant sexual dysfunction. Gonadal activity relies on the pituitary input provided by luteinizing hormone (LH) and follicle-stimulating-hormone (FSH). Although a minimum initial hormonal evaluation consists of FSH and total serum testosterone, the concomitant assessment of LH, prolactin, and estradiol permits one to obtain a more comprehensive picture of the endocrine status of the patient (Table 4.3).

4.2.2 Genetic Testing

When nonobstructive azoospermia or severe oligozoospermia (sperm count $<10 \times 10^6$/mL) is present, karyotype assessment and a search for microdeletions of the long arm of the Y chromosome are recommended [17]. When bilateral or unilateral congenital absence of the vas is detected, and in the presence of obstructive azoospermia or severe oligozoospermia (sperm count $<10 \times 10^6$/mL), screening for CFTR mutations is strongly advised [17]. If anosmia has been identified during medical history taking, and even more so if associated with azoospermia, KAL1 gene screening is recommended, with the aim of detecting the X-linked variety of Kallmann syndrome [18].

4.2.3 Postorgasmic Urinalysis

This test is indicated in men with low-volume or absent ejaculation at orgasm. The presence of any sperm in a postejaculatory urinalysis in these cases is suggestive of retrograde ejaculation.

4.2.4 Specialized Sperm Evaluations

4.2.4.1 Reactive Oxygen Species
Reactive oxygen species (ROS) are generated by both seminal leukocytes and sperm cells; although they have a normal physiological role in capacitation and

acrosome reaction, if in excess they can interfere with sperm function by peroxidation of sperm lipid membranes, and induce DNA damage in both the nuclear and mitochondrial genomes [19]. Chemiluminescent procedures may be used to measure ROS production and the redox activity of human spermatozoa.

4.2.4.2 Sperm Chromatin Assessments

Several methods have been used to test the normality of sperm chromatin and DNA. At present the most used tests are the TUNEL test (terminal deoxynucleotidyl transferase-mediated deoxyuridine triphosphate nick-end labeling], the COMET assay (single-cell gel electrophoresis), and the SCD (sperm chromatin dispersion) test. The results of these tests are correlated with each other [20] and with sperm morphology, motility, and viability [2].

Although sperm chromatin assessments are often advocated in cases of inability to conceive by intercourse, intrauterine insemination, in vitro fertilization (IVF), and IVF using intracytoplasmic sperm injection, it is still controversial as to whether there is any relationship between the results of these tests and the specific reproductive problems [2].

Of note, currently both ROS determinations and sperm chromatin assessments are considered research procedures [2].

4.3 Thinking of the Man, Not Only of the Sperm: Potentials of Infertility Male Workup to Detect Underlying Abnormalities and Risk Factors for Male Health

It has been recently reported that infertile men are overall less healthy than fertile men [21, 22] and that poor semen quality may be a biomarker of general health, associated with worse survival [22].

While the above studies refer chiefly to comorbidities are not typically related to male infertility, two specific conditions more prevalent in infertile men are directly linked to male fertility: testicular germ cell tumors and elevated BMI. Testicular cancer has a 20-fold greater incidence in infertile men than in men with normal fertility [23], and semen parameters of men affected with testis tumor are altered in comparison with healthy controls [24]. Elevated BMI is in turn known to negatively correlate with sperm density [25], sperm motility, and sperm chromatin integrity [26].

Two other risk factors for poor male fertility, namely cigarette smoke [5] and low physical activity [25], though not more prevalent in the infertile male population, are worth mentioning because, along with elevated BMI, they are also well-known cardiovascular risk factors.

The andrologic evaluation of the infertile man has the extra benefit of opening a window on the general health of the man besides his fertility, with the potential to discover life-threatening conditions such as testis cancer, and to identify cardiovascular risk factors which, if corrected, may positively affect the health quality and survival of affected men (Table 4.4).

Table 4.4 Life expectancy, principal conditions, and risk factors more prevalent in infertile men/men with poor semen parameters, versus fertile men

Conditions	Reference
Increased mortality[a]	[22]
Testicular germ cell tumors	[23, 27–29]
Colorectal cancer	[30]
Melanoma	[30]
Prostate cancer	[30]
Cardiovascular disorders	[21]
Pulmonary diseases	[21]
Connective tissue disorders	[21]
Liver diseases	[21]
Diabetes mellitus	[21]
Body mass index	[21]

[a]Increased mortality was due to a wide range of diseases and not particularly diseases related to lifestyle or socioeconomic status

4.4 When to Refer, How to Refer: Key Elements of the Referral Letter

At the conclusion of the andrologic diagnostic workup, the management of the male patient will depend on both the outcome of the workup itself and the possible presence of female infertility risk factors, including advanced female age (>35 years). If a female factor is present, priority should be given to a male treatment strategy that does not delay access to assisted conception programs.

The possible scenarios are summarized in Table 4.5.

As outlined in Table 4.5, a frequent outcome of the andrologic workup is a referral for assisted conception. When this occurs, it is important to write an appropriate referral letter to the assisted reproduction colleagues to adequately summarize the situation regarding the male partner.

Recently, an Italian panel of andrologists and gynecologists proposed a schematic referral letter, aimed to synthetically provide the ART physicians with all the key clinical information concerning the male partner [31]. These five sections of the proposed referral letter are outlined here.

1. *Heading*: This section should report the name and age of both partners
2. *Reason for referral*. This section should summarize the male reproductive history: for how long the man has tried to conceive with the present partner, and possible formerly induced pregnancies (and related outcomes) with the present and, if pertinent, previous partners. Furthermore, results of the male diagnostic evaluation should be summarized: nontreatable male factor infertility versus potentially treatable male factor infertility but suspect/presence of female factor infertility, versus unexplained infertility
3. *Summary of male workup*: Diagnostic conclusions (i.e., varicocele, hypergonadotropic hypogonadism, etc.)

Table 4.5 Management priorities of the infertile couple, according to workup outcomes

MFI	FFI	Management
+, treatable	−	Male treatment + reassessment
+, treatable	+	Male treatment + parallel referral to ART
+, not treatable	+/−	Referral to ART
− (unexplained infertility)	+/−	Referral to ART

MFI male factor infertility, *FFI* female factor infertility, *ART* assisted reproduction treatment

4. *Indications on how to improve sperm quality*: For example, removal of identified risk factors (cigarette smoke, elevated BMI, etc.), specific treatments that may parallel ART (e.g., varicocele correction, genital inflammation treatment)
5. *Special notes, in case of azoospermia*: Type of azoospermia (obstructive vs nonobstructive), results of performed genetic testing, and suggestion on the most appropriate sperm retrieval procedure, in light of the specificity of the case

> **Conclusions**
> Male andrologic workup is mandatory when addressing a couple's reproductive difficulties. The presence of ejaculated sperm, even if sperm values are not below the lower recommended WHO thresholds, should not prevent the male from being evaluated by means of medical history, physical examination, and, possibly, ultrasonography.
>
> Male investigation can allow identification of conditions and risk factors which, when corrected, may improve the chances of both spontaneous conception and success with ART. Furthermore, male andrologic workup may unveil underlying conditions that pose a previously unknown risk for male health.
>
> The extent of male diagnostic investigations must be always appraised in light of the possible presence of female factor infertility.

References

1. Jarow J, Sigman M et al (2010) The optimal evaluation of the infertile male: AUA best practice statement. American Urological Association; Education and Research, Inc, Maryland
2. World Health Organisation (2000) WHO manual for the standardised investigation and diagnosis of the infertile couple. Cambridge University Press, Cambridge
3. Thonneau P, Marchand S, Tallec A et al (1991) Incidence and main causes of infertility in a resident population (1,850,000) of three French regions (1988–1989). Hum Reprod 6:811–816
4. Jungwirth A, Diemer T, Dohle GR et al (2013) Guidelines on male infertility. European Association of Urology. http://www.uroweb.org/gls/pdf/16_Male_Infertility_LRV2.pdf
5. Ramlau-Hansen CH (2007) Is smoking a risk factor for decreased semen quality? a cross-sectional analysis. Hum Reprod 22:188–196
6. Richthoff J, Elzanaty S, Rylander L et al (2008) Association between tobacco exposure and reproductive parameters in adolescent males. Int J Androl 31:31–39

7. Pasqualotto FF (2006) Cigarette smoking is related to a decrease in semen volume in a population of fertile men. Br J Urol 97:324–326
8. La Vignera S, Condorelli RA, Balercia G et al (2013) Does alcohol have any effect on male reproductive function? A review of literature. Asian J Androl 15(2):221–225
9. Toshima H, Suzuki Y, Imai K et al (2012) Endocrine disrupting chemicals in urine of Japanese male partners of subfertile couples: a pilot study on exposure and semen quality. Int J Hyg Environ Health 215:502–506
10. Badawy ZS, Chohan KR, Whyte DA et al (2009) Cannabinoids inhibit the respiration of human sperm. Fertil Steril 91(6):2471–2476
11. Nguyen RH, Wilcox AJ, Skjaerven R, Baird DD (2007) Men's body mass index and infertility. Hum Reprod 22:2488–2493
12. Pauli EM, Legro RS, Demers LM et al (2008) Diminished paternity and gonadal function with increasing obesity in men. Fertil Steril 90:346–351
13. Sharma R, Biedenharn KR, Fedor JM, Agarwal A (2013) Lifestyle factors and reproductive health: taking control of your fertility. Reprod Biol Endocrinol 16;11:66 http://www.rbej.com/content/11/1/66
14. Dubin L, Amelar RD (1970) Varicocele size and results of varicocelectomy in selected subfertile men with varicocele. Fertil Steril 21:606–609
15. World Health Organization (2010) WHO laboratory manual for the examination and processing of human semen, 5th edn. World Health Organization, Geneva
16. Cooper TG, Noonan E, von Eckardstein S et al (2010) World Health Organization reference values for human semen characteristics. Hum Reprod Update 16:231–245
17. Foresta C, Ferlin C, Gianaroli L, Dallapiccola B (2002) Guidelines for the appropriate use of genetic tests in infertile couples. Eur J Hum Genet 10:303–312
18. Franco B, Guioli S, Pragliola A et al (1991) A gene deleted in Kallmann's syndrome shares homology with neural cell adhesion and axonal path-finding molecules. Nature 353:529–536
19. Sawyer DE, Mercer BG et al (2003) Quantitative analysis of gene-specific DNA damage in human spermatozoa. Mutat Res 529:21–34
20. Chohan KR, Griffin TJ, Lafromboise M et al (2006) Comparison of chromatin assays for DNA fragmentation evaluation in human sperm. J Androl 27:53–59
21. Salonia A, Matloob R, Gallina A et al (2009) Are infertile men less healthy than fertile men? Results of a prospective case–control survey. Eur Urol 56:1025–1032
22. Jensen TK, Jacobsen R, Christensen K et al (2009) Good semen quality and life expectancy: a cohort study of 43,277 men. Am J Epidemiol 170:559–565
23. Raman JD, Nobert CF, Goldstein M (2005) Increased incidence of testicular cancer in men presenting with infertility and abnormal semen analysis. J Urol 174:1819–1822
24. Agarwal A, Allamaneni SS (2005) Disruption of spermatogenesis by the cancer disease process. J Natl Cancer Inst Monogr 34:9–12
25. Magnusdottir EV, Thorsteinsson T, Thorsteinsson S et al (2005) Persistent organochlorines, sedentary occupation, obesity and human male subfertility. Hum Reprod 20:208–215
26. Kort HI, Massey JB, Elsner CW et al (2006) Impact of body mass index values on sperm quantity and quality. J Androl 27:450–452
27. Baker JA, Buck GM, Vena JE, Moysich KB (2005) Fertility patterns prior to testicular cancer diagnosis. Cancer Causes Control 16:295–299
28. Doria-Rose VP, Biggs ML, Weiss NS (2005) Subfertility and the risk of testicular germ cell tumors (United States). Cancer Causes Control 16:65–66
29. Eifler JB Jr, King P, Schlegel PN (2008) Incidental testicular lesions found during infertility evaluation are usually benign and may be managed conservatively. J Urol 180:261–264
30. Walsh TJ, Croughan MS, Schembri M et al (2008) Infertile men may have increased risk for non-germ cell cancers: data from 51,318 infertile couples. J Urol 179(Suppl 4):654
31. Pescatori ES, Bartolotti T, Turchi P, Livi C (2013) The andrological referral letter to an assisted reproduction center. Presentation at the course "Infertility: what the Andrologist needs to know" IInd Edition. Zola Predosa (Bologna)

General Therapeutic Approach to Male Infertility

Giorgio Cavallini

5.1 Introduction

The male factor of couple infertility is associated with impaired spermatogenesis in the majority of cases. Because spermatogenesis is a complex process that develops immature stem cells into mature gametes, it is obvious that, independent of the etiology of infertility, there exist harmful agents that are able to exacerbate every cause of infertility. Birth is the intended product of intercourse between a heterosexual couple and subsequent conception, so knowledge of the male partner's fertility conditions is mandatory before an andrologist prescribes any therapy. For this reason a general therapeutic approach to male infertility exists, independent of the cause that generates infertility. This general approach involves evaluation of the therapeutic measures that should be used for all infertile men.

5.2 Sperm Analysis

Male fecundity (defined as the potential male capability to induce pregnancy, independent of female conditions) is related to sperm count. However, this relationship is hyperbolic and achieves a plateau at about 30×10^6 spermatozoa/mL, 50 % class A motility, and 14 % typical forms (strict criteria) [1–3]. Thus in attempting to improve couple fertility, the more severe the dyspermia, the more crucial is its therapy.

G. Cavallini
Andrological Section, Gynepro-Medical Team,
via Tranquillo Cremona 8, Bologna 40137, Italy
e-mail: giorgiocavallini@libero.it

5.3 Female Age

Initially, extensive international data showed fairly consistent age-related risks of Down syndrome live births in different ethnic groups [4]: approximately 1 in 1490 at age 20–24 years, 1 in 200 at 35 years, 1 in 60 at 40 years, and 1 in 11 at 49 years. The observed trisomic births, however, were soon found to be only the tip of the iceberg. Older women have an extremely high rate of pregnancy loss of both chromosomally normal and abnormal conceptions, and increased rates of spontaneous abortions occur at ages similar to those of Down syndrome births. Moreover, spontaneously aborted conceptions that are chromosomally abnormal are mostly trisomic [5].

The reproductive timeline for women is complex. A woman is born with all the oocytes she will ever have, and only 400–500 are actually ovulated [6]. As the number of oocytes declines, a woman's menstrual cycle shortens, infertility increases, and menstrual irregularity begins 6–7 years before the menopause. Increasing age increases a woman's time to pregnancy. When under the age of 30, a woman's chances of conceiving may be as high 71 %; when over 36, it may only be 41 % [7]. The chances of becoming pregnant and being able to maintain a pregnancy are also affected. Matorras et al. reported that in a population of women, the number of infants born begins to exponentially decrease after the age bracket of 35–39 ($n = 89,287$) [8]. The odds of becoming pregnant and maintaining a pregnancy are believed to be connected to numerous factors, including euploidy and dehydroepiandrosterone [9].

These data imply that correction of male fertility should be performed in relation to female age, reserving correction of less severe dyspermias for couples whose female partner is younger than 35 years, with the exception of couples who refuse assisted reproduction. Further correction of dyspermias in couples whose female partner is older than 40 is a non sequitur.

5.4 Diet

Sperm morphology and motility are linked to dietary intake of vitamin C, cryptoxanthin, carotenoid, and lycopene [10, 11]. Consuming a diet rich in carbohydrates, fiber, folate, and lycopene, in addition to fruit and vegetables, correlates with improved semen quality [12]. Consuming lower amounts of both proteins and fats are more beneficial for fertility [13]. In other words, the Mediterranean diet improves male (and female) fecundity [14].

5.5 Smoking Habits

Men who smoke before or during attempts to conceive risk decreasing their fertility (odds ratio 1.6) in comparison with nonsmokers [15]. Men who smoke tend to have a decrease in total sperm count, density, and motility, normal sperm morphology, and semen volume [16, 17]. Smoking may reduce the mitochondrial activity in spermatozoa, and lead to a decreased fertilization capacity [18]. Smoking also can affect the DNA integrity of the sperm, with several studies noting an increase in DNA damage [19].

5.6 Caffeine

It is likely that caffeine intake does not affect spermatogenesis [20].

5.7 Alcohol

In men, alcohol consumption has been linked with many negative side effects such as testicular atrophy, decreased libido, and decreased sperm count [17, 21, 22]. It is likely that sperm count decreases because of a link between alcohol, oxidative stress, and infertility. Oxidative stress has been found to systematically increase with alcohol consumption [23].

5.8 Stress

Stress is defined as mental/emotional tension resulting from a poor/absent compliance to a life situation.

Stress, whether physical, social, or psychological, is a prominent part of any society. Infertility itself is stressful, owing to the societal pressures, testing, diagnosis, treatments, failures, unfulfilled desires, and even fiscal costs with which it is associated [17].

Males who experienced more than two stressful life events before undergoing infertility treatment were more likely to be classified below World Health Organization standards for sperm concentration, motility, and morphology [24]. Stress has a significant impact on sperm density, total sperm count, forward motility, morphology, and DNA fragmentation [24, 25]. Stress and depression are thought to reduce testosterone and luteinizing hormone pulsing [24, 26]. Coping with various lifestyles also affects fertility. It was reported that actively coping with stress, such as being assertive or confrontational, may negatively affect fertility. These data indicate that planning sex in accordance with ovulation day(s) should be ruled out [27–29].

5.9 Exercise

Physically active men who exercised at least three times a week for 1 h typically scored higher in almost all sperm parameters in comparison with those who participated in more frequent and rigorous exercise [30, 31].

5.10 Illicit Drugs

Studies of the effects of illegal drugs on human fertility have been scarce because of ethical considerations, and also subject to under-reporting and bias attributable to the characteristics of the population being studied, such as low socioeconomic status or improper prenatal care [32]. The use of illicit drugs appears to have a negative impact on fertility.

5.10.1 Marijuana

Marijuana acts both centrally and peripherally to cause abnormal reproductive function. Marijuana contains cannabinoids, which bind to receptors located on the vas deferens and inhibit its motility. In males, cannabinoids have been reported to reduce testosterone released from Leydig cells, modulate apoptosis of Sertoli cells, decrease spermatogenesis, decrease sperm motility, decrease sperm capacitation, and decrease acrosome reaction [33].

5.10.2 Cocaine

Cocaine is a stimulant of both the peripheral and central nervous systems that causes vasoconstriction and anesthetic effects. It is thought to prevent the reuptake of neurotransmitters [34], possibly affecting behavior and mood. Long-term users of cocaine claim that it can decrease sexual stimulation; men found it harder to achieve and maintain erection and to ejaculate [35]. Cocaine has been demonstrated to adversely affect spermatogenesis, which may be due to increases in serum prolactin and decreases in serum total and free testosterone [36, 37].

5.10.3 Opiates

Opiates represent another large group of illicit drugs. Opiates such as methadone and heroin are depressants that cause both sedation and decreased pain perception by influencing neurotransmitters. In men taking heroin, sexual function became abnormal and remained so even after cessation [38]. Sperm parameters, most noticeably motility, also decrease with the use of heroin and methadone [37, 39].

5.11 Radiofrequency Electromagnetic Waves (Cell Phones)

Several studies demonstrate negative effects of radiofrequency electromagnetic waves generated by cell phones on sperm count. Cell phone usage has been linked with decreases in progressive motility of sperm, decreases in sperm viability, increases in reactive oxygen species, increases in abnormal sperm morphology, and decreases in sperm counts [40–42]. One study evaluating 52 men demonstrated that those who carried a cell phone around the belt line or hip region were more likely to have decreased sperm motility in comparison with those who carried their cell phones elsewhere or did not carry one at all [42].

5.12 Male Fertility and Longevity

Stress, alcohol, prohibited drugs, smoking habit, Mediterranean diet, and physical exercise are all linked to life expectancy and sperm count. This chapter elucidates why sperm quality can be used as an index of good health and longevity in males [43].

5.13 Residual Fertility

Residual fertility is defined as the probability of a couple to conceive after a period of desiring a child. The longer the period, the lower is the residual fertility (ie, possibility to conceive naturally), even in the case of a correct therapeutic approach and an increase in sperm count [44].

References

1. Bonde JP, Ernst E, Jensen TK, Hjollund NH, Kolstad H, Henriksen TB, Scheike T, Giwercman A, Olsen J, Skakkebaek NE (1998) Relation between semen quality and fertility: a population-based study of 430 first-pregnancy planners. Lancet 352:1172–1177
2. Guzick DS, Overstreet JW, Factor-Litvak P, Brazil CK, Nakajima ST, Coutifaris C, Carson SA, Cisneros P, Steinkampf MP, Hill JA, Xu D, Vogel DL, National Cooperative Reproductive Medicine Network (2001) Sperm morphology, motility, and concentration in fertile and infertile men. N Engl J Med 345:1388–1393
3. Cooper TG, Noonan E, von Eckardstein S, Auger J, Baker HW, Behre HM, Haugen TB, Kruger T, Wang C, Mbizvo MT, Vogelsong KM (2010) World Health Organization reference values for human semen characteristics. Hum Reprod Update 16:231–245
4. Carothers AD, Castilla EE, Dutra MG, Hook EB (2001) Search for ethnic, geographic, and other factors in the epidemiology of Down syndrome in South America: analysis of data from the ECLAMC project, 1967–1997. Am J Med Genet 103:149–156
5. Hassold TJ, Jacobs PA (1984) Trisomy in man. Annu Rev Genet 18:69–97
6. Kimberly L, Case A, Cheung AP, Sierra S, AlAsiri S, Carranza-Mamane B, Case A, Dwyer C, Graham J, Havelock J (2012) Advanced reproductive age and fertility. Int J Gynaecol Obstet 117:95–102
7. Mutsaerts MA, Groen H, Huiting HG, Kuchenbecker WK, Sauer PJ, Land JA, Stolk RP, Hoek A (2012) The influence of maternal and paternal factors on time to pregnancy–a Dutch population-based birth-cohort study: the GECKO Drenthe study. Hum Reprod 27:583–593
8. Matorras R, Matorras F, Exposito A, Martinez L, Crisol L (2011) Decline in human fertility rates with male age: a consequence of a decrease in male fecundity with aging? Gynecol Obstct Invest 71:229–235
9. Ford JH (2013) Reduced quality and accelerated follicle loss with female reproductive aging – does decline in theca dehydroepiandrosterone (DHEA) underlie the problem? J Biomed Sci 13:93

10. Zareba P, Colaci DS, Afeiche M, Gaskins AJ, Jørgensen N, Mendiola J, Swan SH, Chavarro JE (2013) Semen quality in relation to antioxidant intake in a healthy male population. Fertil Steril 100:1572–1579
11. Mínguez-Alarcón L, Mendiola J, López-Espín JJ, Sarabia-Cos L, Vivero-Salmerón G, Vioque J, Navarrete-Muñoz EM, Torres-Cantero AM (2012) Dietary intake of antioxidant nutrients is associated with semen quality in young university students. Hum Reprod 27:2807–2814
12. Mendiola J, Torres-Cantero AM, Vioque J, Moreno-Grau JM, Ten J, Roca M, Moreno-Grau S, Bernabeu R (2010) A low intake of antioxidant nutrients is associated with poor semen quality in patients attending fertility clinics. Fertil Steril 93:1128–1133
13. Wong WY, Zielhuis GA, Thomas CM, Merkus HM, Steegers-Theunissen RP (2013) New evidence of the influence of exogenous and endogenous factors on sperm count in man. Eur J Obstet Gynecol Reprod Biol 110:49–54
14. Vujkovic M, de Vries JH, Lindemans J, Macklon NS, van der Spek PJ, Steegers EA, Steegers-Theunissen RP (2010) The preconception Mediterranean dietary pattern in couples undergoing in vitro fertilization/intracytoplasmic sperm injection treatment increases the chance of pregnancy. Fertil Steril 94:2096–2101
15. Augood C, Duckitt K, Templeton AA (1998) Smoking and female infertility: a systematic review and meta-analysis. Hum Reprod 13:1532–1539
16. Mitra A, Chakraborty B, Mukhopadhay D, Pal M, Mukherjee S, Banerjee S, Chaudhuri K (2012) Effect of smoking on semen quality, FSH, testosterone level, and CAG repeat length in androgen receptor gene of infertile men in an Indian city. Syst Biol Reprod Med 58:255–262
17. Li Y, Lin H, Li Y, Cao J (2011) Association between socio-psycho-behavioral factors and male semen quality: systematic review and meta-analyses. Fertil Steril 95:116–123
18. Calogero A, Polosa R, Perdichizzi A, Guarino F, La Vignera S, Scarfia A, Fratantonio E, Condorelli R, Bonanno O, Barone N (2009) Cigarette smoke extract immobilizes human spermatozoa and induces sperm apoptosis. Reprod Biomed Online 19:564–571
19. Viloria T, Garrido N, Fernandez JL, Remohi J, Pellicer A, Meseguer M (2007) Sperm selection by swim-up in terms of deoxyribonucleic acid fragmentation as measured by the sperm chromatin dispersion test is altered in heavy smokers. Fertil Steril 88:523–525
20. Curtis KM, Savitz DA, Arbuckle TE (1997) Effects of cigarette smoking, caffeine consumption, and alcohol intake on fecundability. Am J Epidemiol 146:32–41
21. Muthusami KR, Chinnaswamy P (2005) Effect of chronic alcoholism on male fertility hormones and semen quality. Fertil Steril 84:919–924
22. Donnelly GP, McClure N, Kennedy MS, Lewis SE (1999) Direct effect of alcohol on the motility and morphology of human spermatozoa. Andrologia 31:43–47
23. Cederbaum AI, Lu Y, Wu D (2009) Role of oxidative stress in alcohol-induced liver injury. Arch Toxicol 83:519–548
24. Gollenberg AL, Liu F, Brazil C, Drobnis EZ, Guzick D, Overstreet JW, Redmon JB, Sparks A, Wang C, Swan SH (2010) Semen quality in fertile men in relation to psychosocial stress. Fertil Steril 93:1104–1111
25. Vellani E, Colasante A, Mamazza L, Minasi MG, Greco E, Bevilacqua A (2013) Association of state and trait anxiety to semen quality of in vitro fertilization patients: a controlled study. Fertil Steril 99:1565–1572
26. Schweiger U, Deuschle M, Weber B, Körner A, Lammers C, Schmider J, Gotthardt U, Heuser I (1999) Testosterone, gonadotropin, and cortisol secretion in male patients with major depression. Psychosom Med 61:292–296
27. Pook M, Tuschen-Caffier B, Kubek J, Schill W, Krause W (2005) Personality, coping and sperm count. Andrologia 37:29–35
28. Volgsten H, Skoog Svanberg A, Ekselius L, Lundkvist O, Sundstrom Poromaa I (2008) Prevalence of psychiatric disorders in infertile women and men undergoing in vitro fertilization treatment. Hum Reprod 23:2056–2063
29. Zorn B, Auger J, Velikonja V, Kolbezen M, Meden-Vrtovec H (2008) Psychological factors in male partners of infertile couples: relationship with semen quality and early miscarriage. Int J Androl 31:557–564

30. Vaamonde D, Da Silva-Grigoletto ME, Garcia-Manso JM, Vaamonde-Lemos R, Swanson RJ, Oehninger SC (2009) Response of semen parameters to three training modalities. Fertil Steril 92:1941–1946
31. Wise LA, Cramer DW, Hornstein MD, Ashby RK, Missmer SA (2011) Physical activity and semen quality among men attending an infertility clinic. Fertil Steril 95:1025–1030
32. Anderson K, Niesenblat V, Norman R (2010) Lifestyle factors in people seeking infertility treatment – a review. Aust N Z J Obstet Gynaecol 50:8–20
33. Battista N, Pasquariello N, Di Tommaso M, Maccarrone M (2008) Interplay between endocannabinoids, steroids and cytokines in the control of human reproduction. J Neuroendocrinol 20:82–89
34. Gold MS, Miller NS (1997) Cocaine and crack: neurobiology. In: Gold MS (ed) Substance abuse: a comprehensive textbook, 3rd edn. Williams & Wilkins, Baltimore, pp 195–218
35. Gold MS (1997) Cocaine and crack: clinical aspects. In: Gold MS (ed) Substance abuse: a comprehensive textbook, 3rd edn. Baltimore, Williams & Wilkins, pp 218–263
36. George VK, Li H, Teloken C, Grignon DJ, Lawrence WD, Dhabuwala CB (1996) Effects of long-term cocaine exposure on spermatogenesis and fertility in peripubertal male rats. J Urol 155:327–331
37. Ragni G, de Lauretis L, Bestetti O, Sghedoni D, Aro VGA (1988) Gonadal function in male heroin and methadone addicts. Int J Androl 11:93–100
38. Wang C, Chan V, Yeung RT (1978) The effect of heroin addiction on pituitary-testicular function. Clin Endocrinol (Oxf) 9:455–461
39. Ragni G, De Lauretis L, Gambaro V, Di Pietro R, Bestetti O, Recalcati F, Papetti C (1985) Semen evaluation in heroin and methadone addicts. Acta Eur Fertil 16:245–249
40. Agarwal A, Deepinder F, Sharma RK, Ranga G, Li J (2008) Effect of cell phone usage on semen analysis in men attending infertility clinic: an observational study. Fertil Steril 89:124–128
41. Agarwal A, Desai NR, Makker K, Varghese A, Mouradi R, Sabanegh E, Sharma R (2009) Effects of radiofrequency electromagnetic waves (RF-EMW) from cellular phones on human ejaculated semen: an in vitro pilot study. Fertil Steril 92:1318–1325
42. Kilgallon SJ, Simmons LW (2005) Image content influences men's semen quality. Biol Lett 1:253–255
43. Omu AE (2013) Sperm parameters: paradigmatic index of good health and longevity. Med Princ Pract 22:30–42
44. Al-Ghazo MA, Ghalayini IF, al-Azab RS, Bani-Hani I, Daradkeh MS (2011) Does the duration of infertility affect semen parameters and pregnancy rate after varicocelectomy? A retrospective study. Int Braz J Urol 37:745–750

Azoospermia

Giorgio Franco, Leonardo Misuraca, and Gabriele Tuderti

6.1 Definition

Azoospermia is defined as the complete absence of sperm in the ejaculate even after centrifugation. Yet even a patient with rare nemasperms after centrifugation in the seminal fluid test is erroneously considered *azoospermic*. This latter condition is instead more correctly defined as *cryptozoospermia*. Instead, severe *oligospermia* is considered a sperm count less than 5 millions/ml. *Azoospermia* must also be differentiated from *aspermia*, which is, instead, the complete absence of seminal fluid emission during orgasm. In this situation the causes are very different and depend on defects of the bladder neck and urethral and ejaculatory ducts system (retrograde ejaculation, urethral stricture, neurological alterations) [1].

6.2 Epidemiology and Classification

Approximately 15 % of couples are unable to procreate after a year of unprotected intercourses and are therefore defined *infertile*. An isolated male factor is present in about 20–30 % of these cases, while in another 20–30 %, there is an association between the male and female factors [2]. Therefore, approximately in half of the cases of couple infertility is the male factor present. The prevalence of azoospermia is approximately 1 % among the general male population and ranges between 10 and 15 % among infertile men [3].

The different types of azoospermia are commonly classified in two large groups: obstructive azoospermia (OA) caused by an obstruction of the passage of sperm

G. Franco (✉) • L. Misuraca • G. Tuderti
Department of Gynecological-Obstetrical and Urological Sciences, Sapienza,
University of Rome, Viale del Policlinico, Rome 00163, Italy
e-mail: giorgio.franco@libero.it; leonardo.misuraca@gmail.com;
gabriele.tuderti@gmail.com

along the seminal pathways and secretory or non-obstructive azoospermia (NOA) due to a sperm production deficit. The latter can then be subdivided into pre-testicular and testicular according to whether the problem derives from an alteration of the hypophisary hormonal system which stimulates spermatogenesis (very rare condition) or from damage intrinsic to the testis (more frequent condition). The prevalence of OA and NOA regarding the total of the different types of azoospermia is very variable according to authors and geographical areas. In countries or cultures where vasectomy is very diffused as a contraception system, a prevalence of slightly higher OA (40 %) [4] can be seen compared to countries, like Italy, where this is rarely done (25–30 %) (Franco G. 2008, unpublished data). It is clear, therefore, that on the whole, the NOAs constitute the majority of the different types of azoospermia (60–75 %). As will be seen in this chapter, even OA and NOA prognosis is rather different and more favourable to OA.

6.3 Aetiology

6.3.1 Obstructive Azoospermia

Obstructive azoospermia is usually classified according to the location of the obstruction (Table 6.1).

6.3.1.1 Testicular Obstruction
The isolated form, with total absence of spermatozoa in the epididymis and normal spermatogenesis, is an extremely rare condition, more often due to a congenital malformation (complete detachment of testicle from epididymis, vasa efferentia and rete testis atresia). The form associated with patchy epididymal obstruction with the presence of some epididymal tubules containing spermatozoa is more frequent and usually due to an acquired post-phlogistic base.

6.3.1.2 Epididymal Obstruction
Obstruction usually happens in the epididymis. It affects about 30–67 % of azoospermic men with normal serum FSH values. The congenital form of it most often appears as bilateral agenesis of the vas deferens (CBAVD), which is associated with a cystic fibrosis gene mutation in 82 % of cases. This form is often correlated to the absence of the distal part of the epididymis (body and tail) and to the agenesis or atresia of the seminal vesicles. Other congenital forms include Young's syndrome which

Table 6.1 Obstructive azoospermia: obstruction location

Testicular obstruction (often congenital, extremely rare)
Epididymal obstruction (post-flogistic, postvasectomy, congenital, Young's syndrome)
Vas deferens obstruction (congenital: partial or complete aplasia; iatrogenic: vasectomy, hernioplasty)
Ejaculatory duct obstruction (cysts, post-flogistic stenosis)

typically is associated with chronic pulmonary infections, normal spermatogenesis and dilation of the head of the epididymis which is full of spermatozoa and amorphous matter, with the absence of spermatozoa in the epididymal corpus region. Among the acquired forms, the most frequent are the obstructions from sexually transmitted infections (gonococcus, chlamydia) and the postvasectomy obstructions from blow-out of the epididymal tubule due to secondary hyperpressure.

6.3.1.3 Vas Deferens Obstruction

The most common cause of congenital obstruction is vas deferens agenesis, almost always associated with the cystic fibrosis gene mutations. In Italy, it has been calculated that about one out of three cases of obstructive azoospermia is caused by vas deferens agenesis. The most frequent form is the complete bilateral one in which the vas cannot be palpated by physical examination, but conditions of partial or unilateral atresia can be observed in which at least one vas deferens or a section of it can be palpated. Unilateral complete or partial aplasia is associated with irregularities of the ejaculatory ducts with to contralateral renal ageneses in 80 and 26 % of cases, respectively.

In the countries where vasectomy is widespread, the most common cause of acquired obstruction is represented by vasectomy as a contraception method. In the United States, almost 500,000 vasectomies are performed per year and approximately 2–6 % of the patients require a conversion (from 10 to 30 thousand reversals/year). In Italy, vasectomy is rarely used; therefore, it is a very less frequent cause of obstruction. Even inguinal hernioplastic surgery can induce vas deferens obstruction via accidental direct damage of it or of its blood supply during surgery. Fibroblastic reaction induced by contact with the polypropylene of the mesh can also determine delayed vas obstruction.

6.3.1.4 Obstruction of the Ejaculatory Ducts

This represents almost 10 % of the obstructive forms of azoospermia and can be congenital (cyst, atresia) or acquired (post-flogistic or dysfunctional).

The utricle, Mullerian and Wolffian cysts are localized in the prostate between the ejaculatory ducts and can be communicating or noncommunicating with the semen pathways and normally cause obstruction by compressive phenomena and lateralization of the ejaculatory ducts themselves. Postinflammatory obstructions, decisively more rare, are secondary to acute, subacute or chronic prostatovesiculitis. When complete, the ejaculatory duct obstructions are associated with a reduced volume of seminal fluid (<1.5 ml) with reduction or absence of fructose, acid pH and dilatation of the seminal vesicles.

6.3.2 Non-obstructive Azoospermia

The non-obstructive forms of azoospermia (secretory) are usually classified according to their cause (Table 6.2). In almost all cases, the cause is at the gonad level (*testicular cause*), while very rarely, only in the case of hypogonadotropic hypogonadism is

Table 6.2 Non-obstructive forms of azoospermia: aetiological classification

1. Idiopathic
2. Genetic
3. Cryptorchidism
4. Testicular torsion
5. Orchitis (viral or bacterial)
6. Varicocele
7. Chemo- or radiotherapy, medicines, toxics
8. Hypogonadotropic hypogonadism

azoospermia attributed to an alteration of the hypophisary gonadotropin secretion (*pre-testicular cause*).

6.3.2.1 Idiopathic

Unfortunately, in almost half of the non-obstructive types of azoospermia, it is difficult to pinpoint the cause connected to the condition, and therefore we speak about an idiopathic or unknown cause. Many of these situations probably have a base of genetic defects which are still unknown, congenital aberrations or a previous unknown exposition to gonadotoxins.

6.3.2.2 Genetic

Karyotype aberrations can be recognized in 10–15 % of azoospermia cases. *Klinefelter's syndrome* is characterized by the presence of a supernumerary X chromosome (47 XXY). One male out of 600 is affected. The patients manifest small and hard testicles, gynecomastia, azoospermia and high levels of gonadotropins. The only possible therapy is testicular sperm extraction (TESE) for intracytoplasmic sperm injection (ICSI). Apparently the best probabilities of success are in younger patients in whom spermatogenesis may not be entirely compromised.

Thanks to recent techniques of molecular biology (PCR), it has been possible to demonstrate that almost 5–10 % of azoospermic patients are a carriers of a *microdeletion of chromosome Y*. This is characterized by alterations of the genes localized in the AZF region (azoospermia factors a, b and c) which have a determining role in spermatogenesis. The complete deletion of the AZFa and AZFb loci is always associated with the absence of spermatozoa in the testicles and therefore with a worse fertility prognosis [5, 6].

6.3.2.3 Cryptorchidism

Cryptorchidism is the undescent of one or both testicles into the scrotum, often linked to a development deficit of the testicles and their ligament connections. In 8 % of cases the testicle remains in the abdomen, in 70 % in the inguinal canal and in 20 % in the pre-scrotum. The greater the degree of retention, the more serious the testicular dysfunction; there is an absence of germinative cells in 20–40 % of testicles in the inguinal or pre-scrotum region and in 90 % of testicles in the intra-abdominal location. In the case of bilateral cryptorchidism, the probability of infertility is 50–90 %, while in the case of monolateral forms, the probability is 20–70 %. Azoospermia caused by cryptorchidism is almost always due to alterations of spermatogenesis connected to the testicular dysgenesis syndrome or due to damage caused by the elevated temperature the retained testicle is exposed to, in particular when not operated on immediately (before 1–2 years of age). Other possible causes of azoospermia are epididymal aberrations often associated with the cryptorchid testicle (didymo-epididymal detachment of testicle from epididymis) which could theoretically cause an obstructive-based azoospermia or mixed secretory-obstructive azoospermia.

6.3.2.4 Testicular Torsion
Testicular torsion can result in azoospermia in the case of bilateral torsion, in monorchid patients or when contralateral testicle is already compromised by other conditions.

6.3.2.5 Orchitis
The parotitis virus can be responsible for orchitis in almost 30 % of affected patients, above all in the post-puberty age, with bilateral interest in 10–30 % of cases. As a result of the infection, an atrophy or permanent testicular hypotrophy can occur with consequent azoospermia. The introduction of the anti-parotitis vaccination has made this event rare. Other bacterial and viral infections or infections from other microorganisms can cause non-obstructive azoospermia from direct damage of spermatogenesis. These germs, however, more frequently cause epididymitis which determine a condition of obstructive azoospermia.

6.3.2.6 Varicocele
The relationship between varicocele and azoospermia is still a matter for discussion. According to most authors, the two conditions could be coexistent only, but for others there is a direct correlation between them. On the basis of this, some suggest the treatment of varicocele which can lead to the reappearance of spermatozoa in the ejaculate, particularly in the presence of a histological pattern of a late maturation arrest or hypospermatogenesis [7].

6.3.2.7 Exposure to Drugs, Toxic Substances and Radiation
Chemotherapy can exercise a negative effect on spermatogenesis. The most affected cells are the spermatogonia and spermatocytes up to the preleptotene stage. The type of drug, its dosage and patient age at time of treatment assume a relevant importance. It seems that alkylating agents and procarbazine are the most toxic for the testicles. During chemotherapy many patients become azoospermic with elevated levels of serum FSH, but the majority of them recover a normal spermatogenesis months or years afterwards. Instead, in other patients, azoospermia is permanent. Also radiation exposure plays a negative role on spermatogenesis; in fact, spermatogonia and spermatocytes are very sensitive to this. Lastly, many toxic substances can cause a serious reduction in spermatogenesis, leading to azoospermia.

6.3.2.8 Hypogonadotropic Hypogonadism
This is a very rare cause of azoospermia (less than 1 % of cases), even if it is the only condition treatable with medical therapy. In hypogonadotropic hypogonadism

the alterations of the hypothalamus or the pituitary gland compromise the correct release of gonadotropins, determining seminal alterations that extend to cases of azoospermia. The Kallmann syndrome is characterized by hypogonadotropic hypogonadism associated with anosmia. An insufficient secretion of GnRh from the hypothalamus with consequent gonadotropin reduction and secondary testicular insufficiency is recognized as the cause of this syndrome. A delayed puberty is a pathognomonic sign. In this condition testicles are usually very small, under 2 cm in longitudinal diameter. Other pathologic conditions affecting the hypophysis diseases such as ischaemia, tumours or infections can cause hypogonadotropic hypogonadism. The Prader-Willi syndrome is characterized by hypogonadism, obesity, muscular hypotonia, mental retardation, reduced development of hands and feet and short stature. These patients have an FSH and LH deficit caused by an insufficiency of GnRh. Therapy for these types of hypogonadism is pharmacological with administration of gonadotropins sometimes associated with GnRh.

6.4 Diagnosis

A careful and accurate andrological evaluation can immediately pinpoint the genesis of azoospermia: personal history, for example, can reveal previous cryptorchidism, testicle infections (orchitis, mostly from epidemic parotitis) or previous chemo- or radiotherapy treatments.

Particular attention is to be paid to:

- Family medical history (even reproductive)
- Personal reproductive medical history and alterations of the ejaculate
- Pathological personal medical history
    - Congenital aberrations (e.g. cryptorchidism)
    - Inflammatory diseases
    - Traumas
    - Inguinal-scrotal and pelvic surgery
    - Systemic diseases
    - Endocrinopathies
    - Chronic obstructive bronchopulmonary diseases
    - Drugs and chemo- and radiotherapy
    - Environmental and professional exposure to heat sources, radiations and toxics

Physical examination can reveal small testicles (<10 ml) with reduced consistence or eunuchoid look of the patient in NOA, while the presence of a normal testicular volume, or unpalpable vasa, will orient towards OA. Physical examination can also show the presence of a varicocele.

The seminal fluid exam can reveal the nature of OA/NOA via the evaluation of volume, pH and fructose. Serum levels of FSH and inhibin B supply further indications for the differential diagnosis between OA and NOA. In fact, an elevated

6 Azoospermia

Fig 6.1 Ultrasound-guided transperineal vesiculodeferentography with fine needle puncture of a median prostatic cysts communicating with the seminal tract

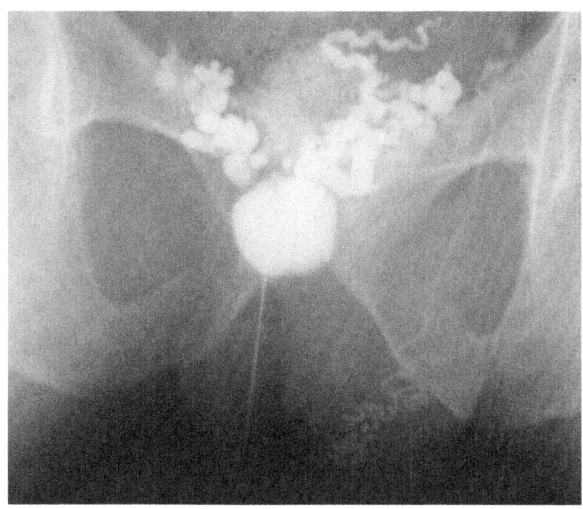

FSH value and a low inhibin B value certainly point to a NOA condition. Scrotum ultrasounds must always be done for the study of the testicle (volume, echogenicity) and epididymis (cribriform pattern suspect for obstruction) but also for the screening of testicular tumours, more frequently found in azoospermic subjects and, in general, in the infertile male. Scrotum echo Doppler or colour duplex scanning must be done in the presence of clinically evident varicocele. TRUS (transrectal ultrasound of the prostate) is recommended in cases of oligoposia, when obstruction of the ejaculatory ducts and agenesis of the vas deferens or seminal vesicles are suspected. As concerns genetic screening, karyotype and chromosome Y microdeletions screening must be done when NOA is suspected and in any case before assisted reproductive techniques (ART). On the other hand, cystic fibrosis gene mutations screening is advised for patients with suspected congenital obstruction but also for the partner, in order to verify the risk of development of cystic fibrosis in the newborn. The invasive diagnostic study, instead, is represented by testicular fine needle aspiration, open testicular biopsy and vasography and vesiculography, which can be performed transscrotally or transperineally via ultrasound-guided needle puncture of the distal seminal tract (Fig. 6.1).

6.5 Therapy

6.5.1 Obstructive Azoospermia

In obstructive azoospermia, when possible, recanalization of the seminal tract and restoration of spontaneous fertility are indicated. Obstruction location and characteristics and partner age influence the choice of treatment.

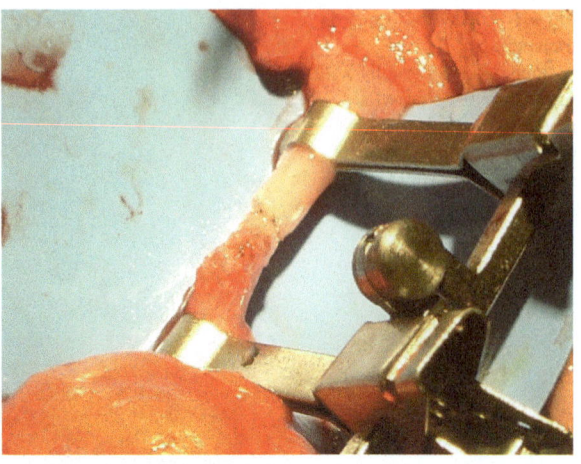

Fig. 6.2 Microsurgical vasovasostomy in two layers according to Silber

- *Microsurgical recanalization of the proximal seminal pathways*
  This treatment is indicated in case of azoospermia, confirmed by at least two recent spermiograms and normal spermatogenesis at least on one side, documented by histology or testicular cytology. Microsurgical reconstruction (epididymovasostomy, vasovasostomy) should be indicated as the first therapeutic option in azoospermia due to epididymal or vasal obstruction. In the majority of patients, it consents the achievement of spontaneous pregnancies by avoiding ART techniques which carry high costs and invasivity to the female partner. In a recent revision of over 4,000 operated cases, Silber reports patency and pregnancy percentages after microsurgical reconstruction at, respectively, 96 and 81 % for vasovasostomy and 84 and 67 % for vasoepididymostomy [8]. The recent introduction of simpler microsurgical anastomosis techniques has further improved results (Figs. 6.2 and 6.3) [9]. When the female partner is older than 37 years, there is, instead, a priority indication for immediate ICSI. This might also be associated with a contextual microsurgical recanalization of the seminal tract.
- *Recanalization of the distal seminal tract*
  Endoscopic resection of the ejaculatory ducts (TURED) or obstructing prostatic cysts is the treatment of choice in distal obstruction. However, its indications have recently been reduced due to the introduction of less invasive techniques and the known possibility of negative postsurgical consequences such as urinary reflux in the seminal tract during micturition [10, 11].

  In the presence of prostatic cysts obstructing the ejaculatory ducts but not communicating with the seminal pathways, a recanalization is possible with a minimally invasive approach of transperineal ultrasound-guided injection and schlerotization of the cysts with alcohol (TRUCA) [10, 11].
- *Sperm retrieval for ICSI*
  When recanalization is not feasible, sperm retrieval and ICSI are indicated [12, 13].

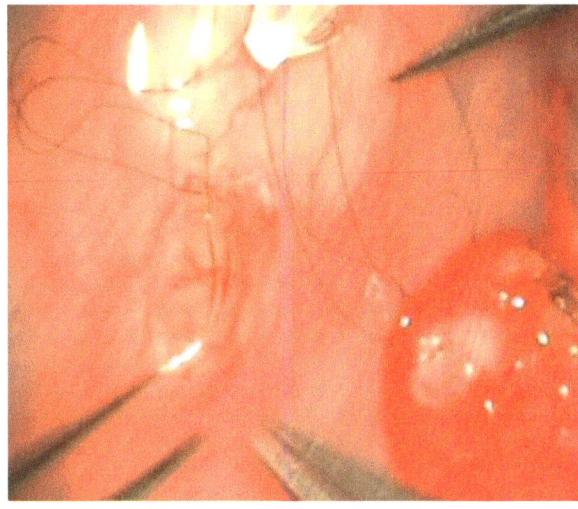

Fig. 6.3 Microsurgical terminolateral vasoepididymostomy (tubulovasostomy): simplified technique with invagination of the epididymal tubule according to Monoski

Table 6.3 Retrieval techniques of male gametes and their acronyms

MESA	Microsurgical epididymal sperm aspiration
PESA	Percutaneous epididymal sperm aspiration
TESA	Testicular sperm aspiration
TESE	Testicular sperm extraction
MicroTESE	Microsurgical testicular sperm extraction

6.5.2 Non-obstructive Azoospermia

Except in the rare cases of hypogonadotropic hypogonadism which can be treated with medical therapy, in patients with NOA the only possible treatment is sperm retrieval for assisted reproductive techniques (ART).

6.5.2.1 Sperm Retrieval Techniques for ART

Sperm retrieval techniques with acronyms are listed in Table 6.3. There is general consensus that in the case of obstructive azoospermia any technique allows a sufficient sperm retrieval for ICSI [14–19]. In fact, by definition, in OA spermatogenesis is normal and sperm can be easily retrieved from the testicle or epididymis even with percutaneous techniques (TESA, PESA) [20, 21]. The original MESA technique is today rarely used because of its high costs and longer surgical times, but its simplification (Mini-MESA), introduced in 1996 [22–24], combines advantages and simplicity of percutaneous techniques with the precision and accuracy of microsurgical procedures. Using a small scrotal incision, the head of the epididymis is exposed and dislocated in the wound, anchoring it at the edges. The procedure continues with the direct puncture of the more dilated and whitish epididymal tubules with a TB syringe (Fig. 6.4). This technique allows one to obtain high counts of sperm and therefore facilitate cryoconservation of an adequate number of paillettes for subsequent ICSI cycles.

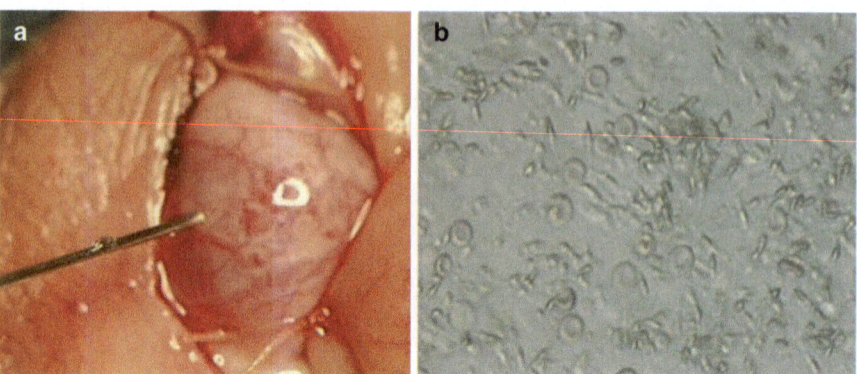

Fig 6.4 Mini-MESA: (**a**) TB needle aspiration from the head of the epididymis, (**b**) sperm retrieval

TESA (or TEFNA, testicular fine needle aspiration) is the simplest percutaneous technique and in OA allows an immediate retrieval of sufficient spermatozoa for one or more ICSI cycles. With a 21G needle butterfly, the testicle is punctured, and with slight movements, testicular fluid is aspirated and sent to the lab for sperm search. PESA is a similar percutaneous technique but performed by inserting the needle into the head of epididymis in order to obtain a more sizeable and clean sperm retrieval compared to TESA. PESA is particularly indicated in congenital absence of the vas deferens. In TESE one or more open surgical biopsies are performed on one or both testicles. TESE is particularly indicated in NOA and when the percutaneous techniques have failed [38].

Many studies have compared ICSI results using freshly retrieved or frozen-thawed sperm, and the majority of these have concluded that there is no difference in terms of fertilization, implantation and pregnancy rates [25].

In NOA the standard treatment is represented by single or multiple TESE [36, 37]. In fact, success rate with percutaneous techniques is extremely low [26, 27]. Overall, in nearly 50–60 % of NOA patients, it is possible to retrieve spermatozoa with TESE [38–40]. Microsurgery has regained interest even in NOA after the introduction of the MicroTESE technique proposed by Schlegel et al. in 1999 [28]. With this technique, many authors have reported a higher rate of sperm retrieval, with less complications compared to multiple TESE [29–31, 36–40]. The technique is performed with an equatorial incision of the tunica albuginea and clam opening of the testicle. Using the magnification of an operating microscope, it is possible to spare the blood supply and to extract single seminiferous tubules with jeweller's forceps. This is done in different areas of the exposed parenchyma, trying to identify the more dilated tubules which more likely harbour sperm (Fig. 6.5).

Extracted tubules are then sent to the laboratory for the search of spermatozoa. The incision is then closed with microsurgical running suture. MicroTESE reduces the possibility of vascular lesions with a lower loss of tissue than multiple TESE. Furthermore, postsurgical pain is reduced due to lesser retraction of the tunica albuginea and consequent less compression of the testicular parenchyma [32].

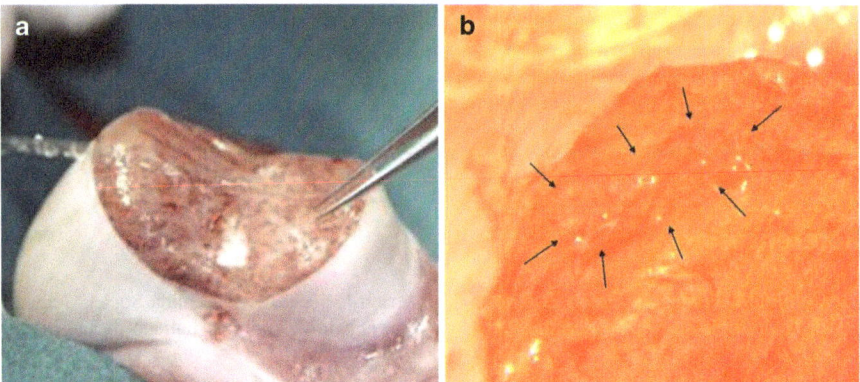

Fig. 6.5 (**a**) MicroTESE: atraumatic extraction of the seminiferous tubule with jeweller's forceps. (**b**) Dilated seminiferous tubules (*arrows* indicate an area of dilated seminiferous tubules)

However, recent reports have shown a reduction in serum levels of testosterone and an increase in LH and FSH after MicroTESE [33].

A New "Stepwise" MicroTESE Approach

Following these considerations, we proposed a "stepwise" approach to MicroTESE in order to reduce invasivity and optimize results, particularly for those patients who did not have previous TESE or histology and whose chance of sperm retrieval is unknown or unclear. Under local anaesthesia (cord block and skin infiltration), a small (10 mm) scrotal window incision is performed and a single testicular biopsy (5 mm) is taken from the mid-portion of the testis and sent to the lab for sperm extraction together with a specimen for histology. If there is presence of sperm, the procedure is terminated and the wound closed. In case of absence of sperm, the scrotal incision is expanded, and the horizontal albuginea incision is also extended equatorially until the testicle is split open and MicroTESE performed. We believe that this approach can optimize the results and reduce the invasivity of sperm retrieval procedures. In fact, although MicroTESE has been shown to be less invasive than multiple TESE [34], a significant hormonal impairment has been described after one or more MicroTESE procedures [33].

Several questions concerning the sperm retrieval techniques in NOA are still being discussed. The possibility of programming the sperm retrieval procedure on the same day of ICSI, in order to use fresh sperm, has been taken into consideration by Verheyen et al. [35]. The authors conclude that there are no significant differences regarding the implant, embryo transfer and pregnancy rate after ICSI with fresh or cryconserved sperm, and therefore they propose, for all patients with NOA, a planned TESE for diagnostic and therapeutic aims, with cryoconservation of the retrieved spermatozoa followed by a differed ICSI. In this way a useless ovarian stimulation of the partner can be avoided in the case of failed sperm retrieval. The superiority of TESE over TESA in NOA has been confirmed by Hauser et al. in a study on the evaluation of the sperm retrieval rate after TESA and multiple TESE in 32 patients with NOA [26, 36–40].

In conclusion, in sperm retrieval techniques, the complexity of the clinical situations and the multiplicity of the therapeutic options presently available suggest the need for a correct evaluation and management of the azoospermic patient. An expert in the field, adequately trained and with competences both in male genital surgery and reproductive medicine, will be able to best carry this out.

References

1. Colpi GM, Franco G, Greco E, Ortensi A, Palermo R (1998) Linee Guida Società Italiana di Andrologia su: l'azoospermia. Parte Prima: la Diagnosi. Giornale italiano di andrologia 5/1:2–13
2. Thonneau P, Marchand S, Tallec A et al (1991) Incidence and main causes of infertility in a resident population (1,850,000) of three French regions (1988–1989). Hum Reprod 6:811–816
3. Jarow JP, Espeland MA, Lipshultz LI (1989) Evaluation of the azoospermic patient. J Urol 142:62–65
4. American Society for Reproductive Medicine (2008) The management of infertility due to obstructive azoospermia. Fertil Steril 90:S121–S124
5. Reijo R, Lee TY, Salo P et al (1995) Diverse spermatogenic defects in humans caused by overlapping, de novo Y deletions encompassing a novel RNA-binding protein gene. Nat Genet 10:383–393
6. Poongothai J, Gopenath TS, Manonayaki S (2009) Genetics of human male infertility. Singapore Med J 50(4):336
7. Kim ED, Leibman BB, Grinblat DM, Lipshultz LI (1999) Varicocele repair improves semen parameters in azoospermic men with spermatogenic failure. J Urol 162:737–740
8. Silber SJ, Grotjan HE (2004) Microscopic vasectomy reversal 30 years later: a summary of 4010 cases by the same surgeon. J Androl 25(6):845–859
9. Monoski MA, Schiff J, Li PS, Chan PT, Goldstein M (2007) Innovative single-armed suture technique for microsurgical vasoepididymostomy. Urology 69(4):800–804
10. Franco G, Gandini L, Ciccariello M, Martini M, Fabbri A, Laurenti C (1995) Trans perineal distal seminal tract sperm aspiration: an alternative treatment to transurethral resection of the ejaculatory ducts? J Urol 153(Suppl):261a
11. Franco G, Leonardo C, Dente D, Iori F, De Cillis A, Cavaliere A, De Nunzio C, Laurenti C (2009) Treatment of ejaculatory duct obstruction: a new algorithm. J Urol 181(4):735a
12. Foresta C, Ferlin A, Franco G, Gandini L, Garolla A, Krausz C, Lenzi A, Sinisi AA (2005) Percorso andrologico: Terapia delle azoospermie ostruttive. In: Foresta C, Lanzone A, Ferlin A (eds) Consensus: iter terapeutico della coppia infertile. Cleup, Padova, pp 258–263
13. Lee R, Li PS, Goldstein M, Tanrikut C, Schattman G, Schlegel PN (2008) A decision analysis of treatments for obstructive azoospermia. Hum Reprod 23(9):2043–2049
14. Palermo G, Joris H, Devroey P, Van Steirteghem AC (1992) Pregnancies after intracytoplasmic injection of single spermatozoon into an oocyte. Lancet 340:17–18
15. Silber SJ, Ord T, Borrero C, Balmaceda J, Asch R (1987) New treatment for infertility due to congenital absence of the vas deferens. Lancet 2:850–851
16. Silber SJ, Nagy ZP, Liu J, Godoy H, Devroey P, Van Steirteghem AC (1994) Conventional in-vitro fertilization versus intracytoplasmic sperm injection for patients requiring microsurgical sperm aspiration. Hum Reprod 9:1705–1709
17. Belker A (1994) The sperm microaspiration retrieval techniques study group. Results in the United States with sperm microaspiration retrieval techniques and assisted reproductive technologies. J Urol 151:1255–1259
18. American Society for Reproductive Medicine (2008) Sperm retrieval for obstructive azoospermia. Fertil Steril 90:S213–S218

19. Hovatta O, Moilanen J, Von Smitten K, Reima I (1995) Testicular needle biopsy, open biopsy, epididymal aspiration and intracytoplasmic sperm injection in obstructive azoospermia. Hum Reprod 10:2595–2599
20. Craft I, Tsirigotis M, Bennet V et al (1995) Percutaneous epididymal sperm aspiration and intracytoplasmic sperm injection in the management of infertility due to obstructive azoospermia. Fertil Steril 63(5):1038–1042
21. Belker AM, Louisville KY, Sherins RJ et al (1996) High fertilization and pregnancy rates obtained by nonsurgical percutaneous needle aspiration of testicular sperm. J Urol 155(Suppl):364A
22. Franco G, Di Marco M, Martini M, Di Crosta G, Laurenti C (1996) A new minimally invasive approach of MESA. Minim Invasive Ther Allied Technol 5(Suppl 1):66
23. Franco G, Rocchegiani A, Di Marco M, Martini M, Presta L, Laurenti C (1996) Un nuovo approccio mini-invasivo di MESA. In: Menchini Fabris F, Rossi P (eds) Andrologia '96. Monduzzi, Bologna, pp 357–361
24. Nudell DL, Conaghan J, Pedersen RA, Givens GR, Schriock ED, Turek PJ (1998) The Mini-Mesa for sperm retrieval: a study of urological outcomes. Hum Reprod 13:1260–1265
25. Oates RD, Dubay A, Harris D et al (1995) Efficacy of Intracytoplasmic Sperm Injection (ICSI) using cryopreserved epididymal sperm: preliminary results. J Urol 153(Suppl):497A
26. Hauser R, Yoghev L, Paz C et al (2006) Comparison of efficacy of two techniques for testicular sperm retrieval in nonobstructive azoospermia: multifocal testicular sperm extraction versus multifocal testicular sperm aspiration. J Androl 27(1):28–33
27. Devroey P, Liu J, Nagy Z et al (1995) Pregnancies after testicular sperm extraction (TESE) and intracytoplasmic sperm injection (ICSI) in nonobstructive azoospermia. Hum Reprod 10:1457–1460
28. Schlegel PN (1999) Testicular sperm extraction: microdissection improves sperm yield with minimal tissue excision. Hum Reprod 14:131–135
29. Tsujimura A (2007) Microdissection testicular sperm extraction: prediction, outcome, and complications. Int J Urol 14:883–889
30. Talas H, Yaman O, Aydos K (2007) Outcome of repeated micro-surgical testicular sperm extraction in patients with non-obstructive azoospermia. Asian J Androl 9(5):668–673
31. Ravizzini P, Carizza C, Abdelmassih V, Abdelmassih S, Azevedo M, Abdelmassih R (2008) Microdissection testicular sperm extraction and IVF-ICSI outcome in nonobstructive azoospermia. Andrologia 40(4):219–226
32. Franco G, Zavaglia D, Cavaliere A, Iacobelli M, Leonardo C, De Cillis A, Petrucci F, Greco E (2009) A novel stepwise approach of microtese in nonobstructive azoospermia. J Urol 181(4):731A
33. Takada S, Tsujimura A, Ueda T, Matsuoka Y, Takao T, Miyagawa Y, Koga M, Takeyama M, Okamoto Y, Matsumiya K, Fujioka H, Nonomura N, Okuyama A (2008) Androgen decline in patients with nonobstructive azoospermia after microdissection testicular sperm extraction. Urology 72(1):114–118
34. Ramasamy R, Yagan N, Schlegel PN (2005) Structural and functional changes to the testis after conventional versus microdissection testicular sperm extraction. Urology 65(6): 1190–1194
35. Verheyen G, Vernaeve V, Van Landuyt L et al (2004) Should diagnostic sperm retrieval followed by cryopreservation for later ICSI be the procedure of choice for all patients with non-obstructive azoospermia? Hum Reprod 19(12):2822–2830
36. Ramasamy R, Padilla WO, Osterberg EC, Srivastava A, Reifsnyder JE, Niederberger C, Schlegel PN (2013) A comparison of models for predicting sperm retrieval before microdissection testicular sperm extraction in men with nonobstructive azoospermia. J Urol 189(2):638–642
37. Pening D, Delbaere A, Devreker F (2014) Predictive factors of sperm recovery after testicular biopsy among non-obstructive azoospermic patients. Obstet Gynecol 123(Suppl 1): 189S–190S

38. Marconi M, Keudel A, Diemer T, Bergmann M, Steger K, Schuppe HC, Weidner W (2012) Combined trifocal and microsurgical testicular sperm extraction is the best technique for testicular sperm retrieval in "low-chance" nonobstructive azoospermia. Eur Urol 62(4): 713–719
39. Kim ED (2014) Using contemporary microdissection testicular sperm extraction techniques, older men with nonobstructive azoospermia should not be deterred from becoming fathers. Fertil Steril 101(3):635
40. Deruyver Y, Vanderschueren D, Van der Aa F (2014) Outcome of microdissection TESE compared with conventional TESE in non-obstructive azoospermia: a systematic review. Andrology 2(1):20–24

Varicocele and Infertility

Giovanni Beretta

7.1 Definition and Classification

Varicoceles are abnormally dilated testicular veins (pampiniform plexus) in the scrotum, normally secondary to internal spermatic vein reflux. This common abnormality has implications such as pain and testicle discomfort, failure of testicular growth, and infertility.

Ambroise Pare defined this anatomic problem in 1550 as a tumor of dilated veins, "a compact pack of vessels filled with melancholic blood" [1]. A modern definition of varicocele is a pathologic dilation of the pampiniform plexus or of the cremasteric venous system that is sufficient to allow a retrograde flow of blood back into the venous system when the intra-abdominal pressure increases. Varicocele is a physical abnormality present in 11.7 % of men with normal semen analysis, 25.4 % of men with abnormal semen [2], approximately 25 % of the normal male population, and up to 40 % of men presenting with infertility; it occurs on the left side in as many as 98 % of patients [3].

The following classification of varicocele is useful in clinical practice:

(a) Subclinical varicocele: Not palpable or visible at rest or during Valsalva maneuver but is demonstrable by scrotal ultrasonography and color Doppler examination
(b) Grade 1: Palpable during Valsalva maneuver but not otherwise
(c) Grade 2: Palpable at rest but not visible
(d) Grade 3: Visible and palpable at rest [4, 5].

G. Beretta
Andrological and Reproductive Medicine Unit, Centro Demetra,
via Della Fortezza 6, Firenze 50129, Italy
e-mail: giovanniberetta@libero.it

7.2 Pathogenesis and Etiology

Presumably because of anatomic differences, varicoceles are much more common on the left side. The left internal spermatic vein empties into the left renal vein. It is much longer (6–8 cm) than the right spermatic vein, which drains into the vena cava. This process is thought to result in increased hydrostatic pressure, causing dilation and tortuosity of these vessels.

Although most men with varicoceles are able to father children, there is abundant evidence that varicoceles are detrimental to male fertility, but the exact association between reduced male fertility and varicocele is unknown. Different theories have been proposed to explain this possible association.

7.2.1 Heat

It has long been observed that even minor fluctuations in temperature can affect spermatogenesis and sperm function.

The scrotum is a temperature regulator for the testes, and varicocele can cause an increase in scrotal temperature and thus impair spermatogenesis. In 1973 Zorgnotti and MacLeod were able to correlate the increase in intrascrotal temperature with impaired testicular function in varicocele patients [6]. Later, Lewis and Harrison (1979) also showed a correlation between varicocele, increased scrotal temperatures, and infertility [7]. Hyperpyrexia can also damage sperm production; this may be the way large varicoceles work, but it is difficult to understand how this could be the modus operandi of smaller varicoceles.

Metabolites. Because a varicocele may be caused by retrograde flow of blood from the renal and adrenal veins, in the left side this may contain toxic substances, perhaps a high concentration of catecholamines. In 1974 Comhaire and Vermeulen found the catecholamine concentration to be higher in the spermatic vein of varicocele than in a control group, implying that catecholamines in the pampiniform plexus lead to chronic testicular vasoconstriction and impaired spermatogenesis [8].

Data on the role of metabolites in the varicocele patient is controversial and inconclusive at present.

Ischemia. When markedly distended, especially in large varicoceles, the pampiniform plexus contains a large amount of venous blood that may be sufficient to impede the arterial input to the testis, lower the partial pressure of oxygen, and cause hypoxia. More work is required to substantiate this theory [9].

DNA damage. Varicocele is associated with increased sperm DNA damage, and this sperm pathology may be secondary to varicocele-mediated oxidative stress. Varicocelectomy can reverse this sperm DNA damage, as shown in several studies [10].

Obstruction of the epididymis. Varicocele, when vary large, may cause partial obstruction of the efferent ductules or of the epididymal duct itself, which can impair maturation of spermatozoa in epididymis and lead to motility disturbances [9].

7.3 Diagnosis

The first step to the diagnosis of varicocele is the medical history and physical examination of the patient in both standing and recumbent positions. Rarely will the male have an abnormal feeling or heaviness in the scrotum or have palpated the veins himself. In general, the classic varicocele will disappear in the lying position owing to venous decompression into the renal vein, whereas the varicocele secondary to cancer invasion of the renal vein will remain because of an anatomic block.

The presence and size of varicocele is most frequently diagnosed on testicular ultrasonographic examination (Fig. 7.1).

The reversal of bloody flow can be demonstrated using the Doppler facility (Fig. 7.2).

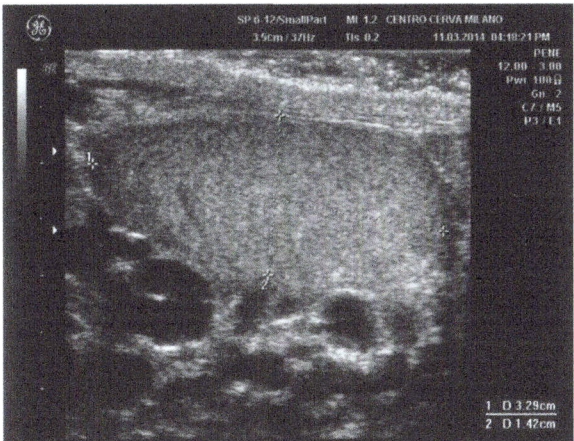

Fig. 7.1 Ultrasonographic appearance of a large left varicocele

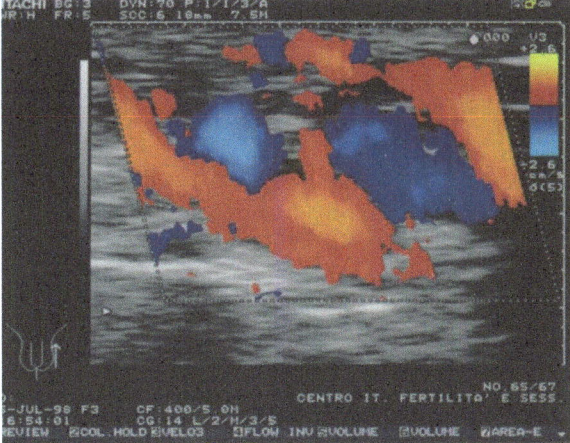

Fig. 7.2 Color Doppler ultrasonogram of left varicocele

Venography is a much more invasive diagnostic method but provides a more detailed view of the varicocele, and also is used to determine the efficiency of a varicocele repair.

Scrotal ultrasonography and color-flow Doppler examination has replaced venography in most cases, and has proved especially useful in those patients so obese that accurate physical examination of the scrotum is impossible.

7.4 Treatment

The clinical benefit of varicocele repair in improving fertility has not been firmly established, but several approaches can be used in the treatment of a varicocele [11].

Open surgery. Open surgical options include retroperitoneal, inguinal, and scrotal approaches, or laparoscopy.

In *the retroperitoneal high procedure* the spermatic vein is ligated at a point above the pelvic brim. With this approach it is not possible to examine any contribution to the varicocele made by the cremasteric venous system. The incidence of hydrocele with this procedure is 5–10 % [12]. Today this procedure is rarely used.

The inguinal approach requires incision in the anterior wall of the inguinal canal and the exposition of the cord; the vas and the artery are identified. Usually there are at least three or four veins that need ligation. There is a high possibility of missing out a branch of testicular vein; some surgeons use a microscope to identify all the vessels in the cord.

The scrotal approach. This procedure produces a very high incidence of hematoma, testicular atrophy, and arterial damage, and is no longer used [13].

Laparoscopy. In this approach the complete vascular bundle is diathermed, and for this reason has many unacceptable complications: injury to testicular artery and lymph vessels, intestinal and nerve damage, bleeding, pneumoscrotum, and wound infection [14].

In general, the risks of surgical varicocele repair are rare and usually mild, and include hydrocele, hematoma formation, wound infections, recurrence of varicocele, and, rarely, testicular atrophy [15, 16].

Percutaneous embolization. This procedure is performed under general anesthesia, is minimally invasive, and is accomplished by embolization of the refluxing internal spermatic vein or veins.

Occlusion of the vein can be performed in a number of different ways such as the use of solid devices, sclerosing agents, and fibrin plugs.

The success of these techniques can be checked by venography [17].

No single method has proven superiority over another as a cure for infertility. On comparing different surgical treatments of varicocele, Al-Kandari et al. showed no clear benefit in favor of any technique in relation to improving sperm parameters [18]. However, the microscopic inguinal approach seems to be associated with significantly less recurrence and potentially fewer complications such as hydrocele, but also requires more operating time and microsurgical training [5].

7.4.1 Medical Treatment

The presence of endocrine dysfunction suggests that certain patients with varicocele and low sperm counts have Leydig cell dysfunction; therefore, human chorionic gonadotropin (hCG) administration might stimulate the testosterone production and the seminiferous tubule activity [19].

Increased numbers of pregnancies have been reported with the use of hCG [20].

Pentoxifylline and antioxidants improve sperm quality in male patients with varicocele. Oliva et al. examined the effect of 12 weeks of daily oral administration of pentoxifylline with zinc and folic acid on the semen quality of 36 men with varicocele-associated infertility in an open, uncontrolled study. After 4 weeks of treatment, the proportion of morphologically normal sperm cells was significantly increased [21].

Although the work presented herein is interesting, the medical treatment in male patients with varicocele remains controversial.

7.5 Discussion

Evers et al. came to the conclusion that clinical evidence supports the concept that there is an association between varicocele and male infertility, but that there is clear evidence showing that appropriate treatment improves a couple's chance of conception [22]. This meta-analysis has been criticized for including several biased heterogeneous studies [23].

Three controlled randomized studies found surgical repair in men with subclinical varicocele to be ineffective [24–26]. Moreover, in men with varicocele and normal semen analysis, no clear benefit has been shown after surgical treatment [27, 28]. For these reasons varicocele repair as a treatment for infertility is not indicated in patients with normal semen parameters or a subclinical varicocele.

In a recent meta-analysis of four randomized controlled studies of varicocelectomy in men with clinical varicocele, oligozoospermia, and otherwise unexplained infertility, a trend in favor of surgical correction was observed [29].

A recent study found an increase in motility of spermatozoa associated with postoperative pregnancy, irrespective of the method by which pregnancy was obtained [30].

However, when the male partner of a couple attempting to conceive has a varicocele, treatment may be considered when all of the following conditions are met:

1. The varicocele is palpable on physical examination of the scrotum
2. The couple has known infertility
3. The female partner has normal fertility or a potentially treatable cause of infertility
4. The male partner has abnormal semen parameters or abnormal results from sperm function tests [31];
5. Varicocele treatment is recommended for adolescents who have progressive failure of testicular development documented by clinical examination [32]

Varicocelectomy improves semen in up to 80 % of infertile men, but the degree of improvement is less clear. In patients with a low sperm count, total motile count varicocelectomy may be of benefit and may reduce the invasiveness of assisted reproductive technologies [33].

Surgical and medical treatment of varicocele is indicated in selected patients with infertility and in others with pain or important local symptomatology [34].

References

1. Hirsch AV, Pryor P (1984) Are there different types of varicocele? In: Glezerman M, Jecht EW (eds) Varicocele and male infertility, vol II. Springer, Berlin, pp 49–52
2. The influence of varicocele on parameters of fertility in a large group of men presenting to infertility clinics. World Health Organisation (1992) Fertil Steril 57:1289–1293
3. Amelar RD, Dubin L (1975) Infertility in the male. In: Karafin L, Kendall AR (eds) Urology, vol II. Harper & Row, New York, pp 19–20
4. World Health Organisation (2000) WHO manual for the standardised investigation and diagnosis of the infertile couple. Cambridge University Press, Cambridge
5. European Association of Urology. Guidelines on male infertility (2012) Eur Urol 62:324–332
6. Zorgnotti AW, MacLeod J (1973) Studies in temperature, human semen quality and varicocele. Fertil Steril 24:854–863
7. Lewis RW, Harrison RM (1979) Contact scrotal thermography: application to problems of infertility. J Urol 122:40–42
8. Comhaire F, Vermeulen A (1974) Varicocele infertility: cortisol and catecholamines. Fertil Steril 25:88–95
9. Glezerman M, Rakowszczyk M, Lunderfeld B et al (1976) Varicocele in oligospermic patients: pathophysiology and results after ligation and division of the internal spermatic vein. J Urol 115:562–565
10. Zini A, Dohle G (2011) Are varicoceles associated with increased deoxyribonucleic acid fragmentation? Fertil Steril 96:1283–1287
11. Nieschlag E, Hertle L, Fischedick A, Abshagen K, Behre HM (1998) Update on treatment of varicocele: counseling as effective as occlusion of the vena spermatica. Hum Reprod 13:2147–2150
12. Wallijn E, Desmet R (1978) Hydrocele: a frequently overlooked complication after high ligation of the spermatic vein for varicocele. Int J Androl 1:411–415
13. Hargrave TB (1994) Varicocele. In: Hargrave TB (ed) Male infertility. Springer, Berlin
14. Tan SM, Ng FC, Ravintharan T, Lim PH, Ching HC (1995) Lararoscopic varicocelectomy: technique and results. Br J Urol 75(4):523–528
15. Johnson D, Pohl D, Rivera-Correa H (1970) Varicocele: an innocuous condition? South Med J 63:34–36
16. Madgar I, Weissenberg R, Lumenfield B, Karasik A, Goldwasser B (1995) Controlled trial of high spermatic vein ligation for varicocele in infertile men. Fertil Steril 63:120–124
17. Seyferth W, Jecht E, Zeitler E (1981) Percutaneous sclerotherapy of varicocele. Radiology 139(2):335–340
18. Al-Kandari AM, Shabaan H, Ibrahim HM et al (2007) Comparison of out-comes of different varicocelectomy techniques: open inguinal, laparoscopic and subinguinal microscopic varicocelectomy: a randomized clinical trial. Urology 69:417–420
19. Weiss DB, Rodriguez-Rigau LJ, Smith KD, Steinberger E (1978) Leydig cell function in oligospermic men with varicocele. J Urol 120:427–430
20. Chehval M, Mehan D (1978) Chorionic gonadotrophins in the treatment of subfertile male. Fertil Steril 31:666–668

21. Oliva A, Dotta A, Multigner L (2009) Pentoxifylline and antioxidants improve sperm quality in male patients with varicocele. Fertil Steril 91(4 Suppl):1536–1539
22. Evers JH, Collins J, Clarke J (2004) Surgery or embolisation for varicoceles in subfertile men. Cochrane Database Syst Rev (3):CD000479
23. Ficarra V, Cerruto MA, Liguori G et al (2006) Treatment of varicocele in subfertile men: the Cochrane review—a contrary opinion. Eur Urol 49:258–263
24. Grasso M, Lania M, Castelli M et al (2000) Lowgrade left varicocoele in patients over 30 years old: the effect of spermatic vein ligation on fertility. BJU Int 85:305–307
25. Yamamoto M, Hibi H, Hirata Y et al (1996) Effect of varicocoelectomy on sperm parameters and pregnancy rates in patients with subclinical varicocele: a randomized prospective controlled study. J Urol 155:1636–1638
26. Unal D, Yeni E, Verit A et al (2001) Clomiphene citrate versus varicocoelectomy in treatment of subclinical varicocoele: a prospective randomized study. Int J Urol 8:227–230
27. Nilsson S, Edvinsson A, Nilsson B (1979) Improvement of semen and pregnancy rate after ligation and division of the internal spermatic vein: fact or fiction? Br J Urol 51:591–596
28. Breznik R, Vlaisavljevic V, Borko E (1993) Treatment of varicocoele and male fertility. Arch Androl 30:157–160
29. Baazeem A, Belzile E, Ciampi A et al (2011) Varicocele and male factor infertility treatment: a new meta-analysis and review of the role of varicocele repair. Eur Urol 60:796–808
30. Baker K, McGill J, Sharma R, Agarwal A, Sabanegh E Jr (2013) Pregnancy after varicocelectomy: impact of postoperative motility and DFI. Urology 81(4):760–766
31. Giagulli VA, Carbone MD (2011) Varicocele correction for infertility: which patients to treat? Int J Androl 34:236–241
32. Paduch DA, Niedzielski J (1997) Repair versus observation in adolescent varicocele: a prospective study. J Urol 158(3Pt 2):1128–1132
33. Samplaski MK, Zini A, Lo KC, Grober ED, Jarvi KA (2013) Varicocelectomy to "upgrade" semen quality to allow couples to use less invasive forms of assisted reproductive technologies. Fertil Steril 100(3):supplement S5
34. Cavallini G, Beretta G, Biagiotti G, Mallus R., Maretti C, Pescatori E, Paulis G. Subsequent impaired fertility (with or without sperm worsening) in men who have fathered children after a left varicocelectomy: a novel population. Urol Ann (in press)

Chromosomic Causes of Infertility

Gianni Paulis

8.1 Definition and Epidemiology

The main genetic factors involved in male infertility are chromosomal abnormalities. These abnormalities can be structural (e.g., deletions, duplications, translocations, inversions, etc.) or numerical (e.g., trisomy, tetrasomy, aneuploidy, etc.) [1, 2] and involve sex chromosomes (e.g., Klinefelter syndrome, 47,XXY) or autosomes (reciprocal translocations and Robertsonian translocations). The incidence of chromosomal aberrations in the general population is approximately 0.5–0.6 % [3–6]. About 1 in 150 babies is born with a chromosomal abnormality [7, 8]. Chromosomal abnormalities account for about 5 % of infertility in males, and the prevalence reaches approximately 15–20 % of the azoospermic males [9, 10] and 5–10 % of the oligozoospermic males [11]. Karyotype abnormalities are reported in 2–14 % of males presenting with infertility [12]. Klinefelter syndrome and Y-chromosomal microdeletions are the most frequent genetic cause of male infertility.

8.2 Etiology

Chromosomal abnormalities are caused by *errors in the number or structure of chromosomes*. It is still unknown why these errors occur.

The *errors in the number of chromosomes* occur during cell division (mitosis and meiosis).

A chromosomal abnormality can also occur before fertilization.

Meiosis is the process of division of reproductive cells (with half the number of chromosomes, 23, haploid cell): eggs and sperms.

G. Paulis
Department of Urology, Andrology Center, Regina Apostolorum Hospital,
Via S. Francesco, 50, Rome, Albano Laziale 00041, Italy
e-mail: paulisg@libero.it

If this process does not occur properly, the chromosomes do not segregate properly, and gametes, eggs, or sperms may end up with too few (monosomy) [13] or too many chromosomes (trisomy) [14].

Errors can also occur during mitosis, after fertilization, when the chromosomes are being duplicated during fetal development resulting in mosaicism: some cells with a typical number of chromosomes and some with an incorrect number of chromosomes.

The *errors in structure of chromosomes* can occur, usually before fertilization, and change the structure of one or more chromosomes. Usually, individuals with structural chromosomal abnormalities have a normal number of chromosomes, but a portion of a chromosome is missing, deleted or inverted, duplicated, misplaced, or exchanged with another part of another chromosome.

Chromosome abnormalities can be inherited from a parent, such as the translocation, or may also occur for the first time in an individual [15].

An important causal factor of chromosomal abnormalities is the *maternal age* (over 35 years) as the primary risk factor for nondisjunction during meiosis, which leads to the occurrence of trisomy 21 (Down syndrome) [16], trisomy 18 (Edward syndrome) [17], and trisomy 13 (Patau syndrome) [18].

The *paternal age* is less important as a causal factor of chromosomal abnormalities [19–21].

Environmental factors can cause chromosomal aberrations although there are few demonstrations [22–25].

8.3 Pathology, Diagnosis, Therapy, and Prognosis

The majority of human chromosomal abnormalities occur in the autosomes. The most common autosomal abnormalities are trisomy 21 (Down syndrome), trisomy 18 (Edward syndrome), trisomy 13 (Patau syndrome), partial deletion of the short arm of chromosome 4 (Wolf–Hirschhorn syndrome), and deletion of the short arm of chromosome 5 (cri du chat syndrome). Individuals with these autosomal abnormalities usually have multiple physical malformations, mental retardation, and relatively short lives. The most common sex chromosome abnormalities are Klinefelter syndrome, monosomy X (Turner syndrome), and fragile X syndrome. These sex chromosome abnormalities are slightly less common than autosomal abnormalities, and they are generally much less severe in their effects, and the first two are not associated with mental retardation.

However, for the purposes of this chapter the author has chosen to focus mainly on the most common chromosomic causes of infertility [26]:

- Numerical sex chromosome abnormality = 54 %
- Structural chromosomal aberrations: chromosomal translocations (autosomal translocation, 15 %; Robertsonian translocation, 8 %; sex chromosome translocation, 4 %), Y-chromosomal microdeletions, and CFTR gene deletions or duplications
- Others = 19 %

Fig. 8.1 The Klinefelter's distribution

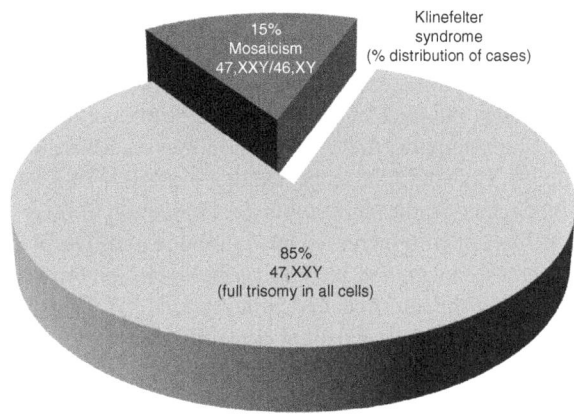

Table 8.1 Klinefelter syndrome

Common clinical signs
Infertility (azoospermia or oligospermia)
Small testes
Hypergonadotropic hypogonadism
Gynecomastia
Tall height
Learning difficulties (children)
Long arms and legs
Shorter torso
Decreased facial and pubic hair (adults)
Psychosocial or behavioral problems

8.3.1 Klinefelter Syndrome (47,XXY)

Klinefelter syndrome (KS) is the most common numerical sex chromosome disorder in males caused by aneuploidy, affecting one in 660 newborn males [27]. This disease was described for the first time in 1942 [28].

KS is usually associated with the karyotype 47,XXY which may be in all cells (full trisomy) or in mosaic form (15 % of the cases, see Fig. 8.1) [29]. In KS mosaicism some of the cells only have an extra X chromosome (47,XXY/46,XY).

The extra X chromosome derives from nondisjunction during meiosis and may have a paternal (>50 %) or maternal (40–50 %) origin [29]; for the rest of the cases, the X chromosome is originated post-zygotically [30]. The only way to confirm the presence of an extra X chromosome is by a karyotype analysis of peripheral blood or on amniocytes or chorionic villi from prenatal specimens. Common signs and symptoms are small testes (bi-testicular volume <6 ml) [31], hypergonadotropic hypogonadism, gynecomastia, learning difficulties (children), azoospermia and decreased facial and pubic hair (adults), long arms and legs, and tall height (see Table 8.1). Most, but not all, patients affected by KS, are infertile with small testicles, increased numbers of Leydig cells, tubular sclerosis, and interstitial fibrosis of varying degrees [32]. The physical manifestations of KS are often variable.

This syndrome generally causes spermatogenesis arrest at the primary spermatocyte stage, but occasionally later stages of sperm maturation are observed [33]. It has been estimated that 25 % of non-mosaic KS patients have sperm in their ejaculate [9]. Paduch (2008) reported that over 50 % of KS patients were not sterile [34]. Some recent studies have reported a reduction of life expectancy for KS patients by 1.5–2 years, with increased mortality due to different disorders: diabetes, lung cancer, breast cancer, non-Hodgkin lymphoma, cerebrovascular disease, vascular insufficiency of the intestine, and epilepsy [35, 36]. Klinefelter syndrome should first be suspected whenever a patient consults the doctor because of infertility. In this case these following tests should always be performed: karyotype analysis, semen count, and blood test to check hormone levels of follicle-stimulating hormone, luteinizing hormone, testosterone, and estradiol. Differential diagnoses for KS may include the following conditions: fragile X syndrome, Marfan syndrome, and Kallmann syndrome. With the introduction of the procedure intracytoplasmic sperm injection (ICSI), which consists of the use of sperm extraction from deep within the testicles of KS patients (non-mosaic), some 47,XXY men will have an increased chance of fathering a child [37–39]. Androgen replacement therapy in KS patients should begin in puberty to promote linear growth and secondary sexual characteristics and to permit the normal accrual of muscle mass, bone mineral content, and the adult regional distribution of body fat [40]. However, this treatment is ineffective for treating infertility, gynecomastia, and small testes. Treatment options include different routes of administration: transdermal, oral, and intramuscular injections. A gradual increase of dosage sufficient to maintain age-appropriate serum concentrations of testosterone, estradiol, FSH, and LH is recommended.

8.3.2 Structural Chromosomal Aberrations

- *Chromosomal translocations*
- *Y-chromosomal microdeletions*
- *CFTR gene deletions or duplications*

8.3.2.1 Chromosomal Translocations
Chromosomal translocations are caused by the rearrangement of parts between non-homologous chromosomes.

There are two types of chromosomal translocations: reciprocal or Robertsonian translocations.

Reciprocal translocations occur when there is an exchange of chromosomal material between two different chromosomes. When translocations affect the non-sex chromosomes, they are called autosomal translocations. These translocations occur in 1 in 500 newborns and are the most commonly observed structural chromosomal anomalies in infertile men [26]. Reciprocal translocations can be inherited from a parent, or they can appear de novo. Translocations are "balanced" when the chromosome material has been rearranged but no genetic material has been lost or gained. Balanced translocations do not usually impact on the growth or development of the individual involved. Nevertheless, carriers (parents) of balanced translocations (who are normal phenotypes) produce both balanced and unbalanced gametes with deletions and duplications of large pieces of the chromosomes involved. The child conceived by an unbalanced gamete inherits a rearrangement of the chromosomes with deletion and/or duplication of chromosome; this condition is known as an unbalanced translocation. Although carriers of balanced chromosomal translocations are phenotypically normal, they may experience reduced fertility, spontaneous abortions, or birth defects [41, 42].

Autosomal translocations negatively affect spermatogenesis due to disrupted meiotic pairing and segregation [43–45]. While translocations have no effect on other tissues, these aberrations can seriously impair spermatogenesis causing severe oligozoospermia or azoospermia [45, 46].

In the same way that occurs in other chromosomal translocations, any part of the sex chromosome may translocate to autosomes. Translocations affecting sex chromosomes have direct consequences on genes involved in spermatogenesis. Translocations between the Y chromosome and autosomes are rare and often cause abnormal spermatogenesis and infertility [47, 48]. The possible mechanisms for reduced fertility due to sex chromosome translocation are the altered gene loci or altered formation of sex vesicle during meiosis.

Translocations involving a sex chromosome and an autosome cause infertility more easily than translocations involving autosomes.

When translocations involve acrocentric chromosomes, these aberrations are called Robertsonian translocations.

Robertsonian translocations involve only these chromosomes and specifically chromosomes 13, 14, 15, 21, and 22. This type of translocation originates from a centric fusion of two acrocentric chromosomes.

When two chromosomes fuse at the centromere (centric fusion), the result is a Robertsonian translocation. Robertsonian translocation is the most frequent structural chromosomal abnormality in humans, and it occurs in around 1 in 1,000 live births [49]. Balanced Robertsonian translocations do not usually impact on the growth or development of the individual involved. Nevertheless, carriers (parents) of Robertsonian translocations, as with reciprocal translocations, can have reproductive effects, when the child receives the translocation in an unbalanced form. Robertsonian translocations can cause various degrees of sperm alteration (oligospermia or azoospermia) [50, 51]. Robertsonian translocations are more common in oligozoospermic and azoospermic men, with rates of 1.6 and 0.09 %, respectively [52].

Robertsonian translocations involving chromosome 21 are found in 5 % of patients with Down syndrome [53].

Preimplantation genetic diagnosis (PGD) by fluorescence in situ hybridization (FISH) is recommended for a Robertsonian translocation and may be useful for couples who opt for assisted reproductive techniques [26].

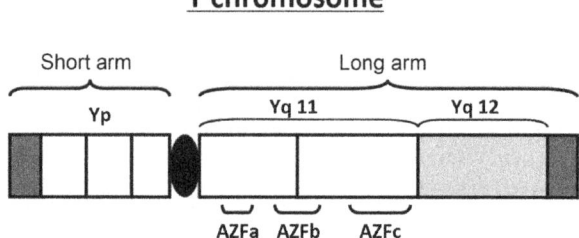

Fig. 8.2 Schematic representation of human Y chromosome

8.3.2.2 Y-Chromosomal Microdeletions (Y Chromosome-Related Azoospermia)

The Y chromosome is the smallest human chromosome and contains many of the genes that are necessary for spermatogenesis and the development of testes. Y-chromosomal microdeletions, which span several genes and remove one or more of them, are able to cause various spermatogenic defects. Y-chromosomal microdeletions are determined by submicroscopic deletions on the Y chromosome (Yq11 region) (see Fig. 8.2), and these alterations are not large and visible by conventional cytogenetic methods. After the Klinefelter syndrome, Y-chromosomal microdeletions are the most frequent genetic cause of male infertility [54, 55]. These gene deletions have been attributed to intrachromosomal homologous recombination within unstable amplicons clustered within the AZF region (azoospermia factor region) [56]. Y chromosome-related azoospermia is the most frequent structural chromosomal anomaly associated with failure in sperm production. The incidence of this anomaly is 15–20 % in men with idiopathic azoospermia and 7–10 % in men with idiopathic severe oligozoospermia [57]. Y-chromosomal microdeletions are extremely rare in infertile males with a sperm concentration >5 million/ml. Generally, Y-chromosomal microdeletions are "de novo" events and are estimated to occur in one in 2,000–3,000 males [58–61]. Infertile men with Y-chromosomal microdeletions usually have no visible symptoms, although some have small testicles and/or cryptorchidism. The first association between azoospermia and deletions of the long arm of the Y chromosome was demonstrated by Tiepolo (1976) [62].

Microdeletions most frequently occur on the long arm of the Y chromosome, Yq 11 region. An important area of interest on Yq is the AZF region that contains genes involved in germ cell development. This region contains three subregions: AZFa, AZFb, and AZFc [63] (see Fig. 8.2).

Gene deletions in this region cause various spermatogenic and infertility phenotypes [64]. Severe infertility or azoospermia is manifest when AZFa, AZFb, or AZFc is singly, or in combination, deleted from the genome. AZFc deletions are the most common form of Y-chromosomal microdeletions and account for approximately 58.3–69 % of reported microdeletions [65–67], followed by deletions of the AZFb region (14 %) and deletions of the AZFa region (6 %) [67]. Zhang et al. reported these incidence rates of several possible combinations of AZF region microdeletions [68]: AZFa = 1.7 %, AZFb = 12.5 %, AZFc = 64.2 %, AZFb + c = 20.0 %, and AZFa + b + c = 1.7 %.

AZFc deletions are usually associated with low levels of sperm in the ejaculate or azoospermia (about two-thirds of individuals) [69]. Transmission of Y-chromosomal AZFc microdeletions could potentially result in the development of sexual ambiguities and Turner stigmata (45,X0) [70, 71]. Microdeletions of AZFa are associated with the complete Sertoli-cell-only (SCO) syndrome and azoospermia, while microdeletions of AZFb or AZFc result in a variable clinical and histological phenotype, ranging from the SCO syndrome to oligozoospermia [72–74]. AZFb+c deletions usually produce no testicular sperm. When AZF-deleted sperms are used for *assisted reproductive techniques* (ART), fertility defects in male offspring are inevitable [65]. Classical Y-chromosomal microdeletions do not confer a risk for cryptorchidism or testicular cancer [74, 75]. If complete AZFa or AZFb microdeletions are detected, micro-testicular sperm extraction (TESE) is not indicated because this technique is very time consuming—it is extremely difficult to find sperm cells [74]. Microdeletion analysis using PCR helps determine the frequency and site of gene deletion and thus the testicular phenotype. Yq microdeletion analysis (AZF screening) is generally carried out by multiplex polymerase chain reaction (PCR) amplifying AZFa, AZFb, and AZFc loci in the q arm of the Y chromosome [76]. The analysis of Y-chromosomal microdeletions permits to establish a diagnosis and to formulate a prognosis, in men with idiopathic infertility presenting with azoospermia or severe oligospermia with sperm concentrations <5 million/ml [77]. AZF screening is important before varicocelectomy because infertile men carrying a Yq microdeletion will most likely not benefit from the surgical procedure [77]. In case of diagnosis of Y-chromosomal microdeletion, a genetic counseling is mandatory (especially for the ART candidates) to provide information about the risk of conceiving a son with impaired spermatogenesis.

8.3.2.3 Mutations in the CFTR Gene

Congenital bilateral absence of the vas deferens (CBAVD) is an important disorder characterized by agenesis of the vas deferens, and it affects about one in 1,000 male individuals [78]. It is an important cause of sterility in men, approximately 2 % of infertility cases [79], and it accounts for 6 % of cases of obstructive azoospermia (OAZ) [80].

Genetic mutations in the cystic fibrosis transmembrane conductance regulator gene (CFTR) are responsible for CBAVD and cystic fibrosis (CF). The CFTR gene is located on the long (q) arm of human chromosome 7 at position 31.2 [81] (see Fig. 8.3).

CFTR gene mutations are responsible in about 95 % of men with CBAVD [82].

Cystic fibrosis is the most frequent severe autosomal recessive genetic disorder in the Caucasian population, affecting about 1 in 2,500 live births [83]. The most frequent clinical manifestations of CF are chronic obstruction and infection of the respiratory tract and often exocrine pancreatic insufficiency. About 98 % of male CF patients are infertile as a result of CBAVD [84, 85]. The CFTR gene encodes for a membrane protein that also influences the formation of the ejaculatory duct, seminal vesicle, vas deferens, and distal two-thirds of the epididymis.

Fig. 8.3 Location of the CFTR gene on human chromosome 7

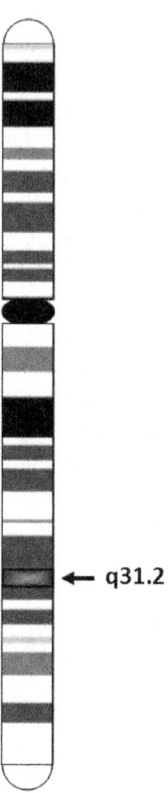

Genetic mutations in the CFTR gene (deletions or duplications) lead to the low function of CFTR resulting in the production of viscous secretions (dehydration of mucus secretions) that obstruct the lumen of airways, sweat glands, gastrointestinal tract, pancreatobiliary ducts, sinuses, and reproductive tissues [86].

CBAVD may also occur as an isolated form of genital disorder without clinical CF symptoms (incomplete genital form of CF) [87]. Patients with this phenotype of CF, previously considered a distinct genetic entity, have an increased frequency of CFTR gene mutations [88, 89]. CFTR gene mutations were detected in some patients with congenital unilateral absence of the vas deferens (CUAVD); this condition could be an incomplete form of CBAVD [89]. CUAVD is a rare condition and has an incidence of 0.5–1 % in the male population [90]. CUAVD was found to occur twice as frequently on the left than on the right side [91]. Whereas in some of CUAVD patients the condition is associated with mutations in the CFTR gene, in other patients this congenital anomaly is probably caused by other factors [88]. Men with CUAVD may be normally fertile [88]; in these males there is a high incidence of ipsilateral renal agenesis [92]. CUAVD is interesting because of its association with renal anomalies and CFTR gene mutations [92]. Renal imaging and cystic fibrosis (CF) screening were recommended to all patients with CUAVD or CBAVD. In fact unilateral renal agenesis is also possible in CABVD patients with an incidence of about 10 %, mostly seen in patients without CFTR gene aberrations [93].

Screening for CFTR mutations is recommended in the following conditions:

- Azoospermic male with a semen volume of < 1.5 ml and pH less than 7.0
- Individuals with a family history of CF or CFTR mutations
- Males with CBAVD or CUAVD
- Patients with chronic or idiopathic pancreatitis
- Reproductively active individuals or couples
- Couples who opt for ART (assisted reproductive techniques) for determining the risk of transmitting CFTR mutations to the offspring

8.3.3 Prader–Willi Syndrome

Prader–Willi syndrome (PWS) is a rare genetic disease which occurs equally in both sexes and all races.

PWS was first described in 1956 [94] and has a prevalence about of one in 50,000 newborns [95–98].

This syndrome is characterized by severe muscular hypotonia, hyperphagia, obesity, hypogonadism, mental retardation, and short stature. This condition is caused by the absence of paternal expression of imprinted genes localized in the 15q11-q13 region [94, 99]. However, the following are possible genetic subtypes [100]: paternal deletion of chromosome 15q11-q13 (type I or II), 75 %; maternal uniparental disomy (UPD), 24 %; imprinting center defects (ID), 1 %; and translocation <1 %.

Delayed and incomplete pubertal development is documented in almost all PWS patients. Manifestations of hypogonadism in infancy include micropenis and/or cryptorchidism (80 %) in males [101, 102]. Hypogonadism was generally considered to be of hypothalamic origin [102–105].

DNA methylation analysis is the only technique, which can both confirm and reject the diagnosis of this syndrome [86]. A prenatal diagnosis could be suspected in cases of reduced fetal movement and polyhydramnios [106]. In a family who previously had a child with PWS (with an imprinting defect), the man with a deletion has a 50 % chance of fathering a baby with PWS again [100]. At present there are no reports of paternity in PWS [100].

A possible therapeutic program should include:

- Obesity management with institution of a low-calorie, well-balanced diet, with regular exercise and rigorous supervision
- GH treatment in children to improve growth during childhood
- Hormonal treatment for induction, promotion, or maintenance of puberty
- Management of behavioral and psychiatric problems

8.3.4 Angelman Syndrome

Angelman syndrome (AS) is a rare condition caused by deletion on the mother's chromosome 15. The incidence is one in 12,000–20,000 births [107–109]. Angelman syndrome is a rare neurological disorder characterized by developmental delay, significant intellectual disability, difficulties with speech development, seizures, uncontrolled limb and body movements, motor impairment, spontaneous laughter, EEG abnormalities, and epilepsy [110]. Anomalies of the head and face are common, including microcephaly, macrostomia, maxillary hypoplasia, mandibular prognathism, deeply set eyes, and widely spaced teeth. Males and females with Angelman syndrome achieve puberty normally, with normal secondary sexual characteristics. However, there has been no documented case of reproduction in a male with Angelman syndrome [110]. A successful reproduction has been reported in only one case of female with Angelman syndrome [110].

DNA methylation analysis identifies approximately 80 % of individuals with AS. If the DNA methylation analysis is abnormal, the next step is FISH or array CGH analysis [111].

For completeness, other very rare forms of male infertility caused by genetic disorders [79] are listed at the end of this chapter:

- Myotonic dystrophy (DM)
- Kallmann syndrome
- Immotile cilia syndrome
- Noonan syndrome
- Denys–Drash syndrome (DDS) and Frasier syndrome
- Androgen insensitivity syndrome
- Polycystic kidney disease (with multiple cysts in the liver, kidneys, epididymis, and seminal vesicles)
- Usher's syndrome

References

1. Johnson MD (1998) Genetic risks of intracytoplasmic sperm injection in the treatment of male infertility: recommendations for genetic counseling and screening. Fertil Steril 70:397–411
2. van Assche EV, Bonduelle M, Tournaye H et al (1996) Cytogenetics of infertile men. Hum Reprod 11(Suppl 4):1–24; discussion 25–26
3. Berger R (1975) The incidence of constitutional chromosome aberrations. J Genet Hum 23:42–49
4. Hamerton JL, Canning N, Ray M et al (1975) A cytogenetic survey of 14,069 newborn infants. I. Incidence of chromosome abnormalities. Clin Genet 8:223–243
5. Hook EB, Hamerton JL (1977) The frequency of chromosome abnormalities detected in consecutive newborn studies; differences between studies; results by sex and by severity of phenotypic involvement. In: Hook EB, Porter IH (eds) Population cytogenetics: studies in humans. Academic, New York, pp 63–79

6. Patil SR, Lubs HA, Brown J et al (1977) Incidence of major chromosome abnormalities in children. Cytogenet Cell Genet 18:3102–3106
7. American College of Obstetricians and Gynecologists (2001) ACOG Practice Bulletin No. 27: Clinical Management Guidelines for Obstetrician-Gynecologists. Prenatal diagnosis of fetal chromosomal abnormalities. Obstet Gynecol 97(5 Pt 1):suppl 1–12
8. Carey JC (2003) Chromosomal disorders. In: Rudolph CD, Rudolph AM (eds) Rudolph's pediatrics, 21st edn. McGraw-Hill Medical Publishing Division, New York, pp 731–741
9. Ferlin A, Raicu F, Gatta V et al (2007) Male infertility: role of genetic background. Reprod Biomed Online 14:734–745
10. O'Flynn O'Brien KL, Varghese AC, Agarwal A (2010) The genetic causes of male factor infertility: a review. Fertil Steril 93:1–12
11. Dada R, Gupta NP, Kucheria K (2006) Cytogenetic and molecular analysis of male infertility: Y chromosome deletion during nonobstructive azoospermia and severe oligozoospermia. Cell Biochem Biophys 44:171–177
12. Shi Q, Martin RH (2000) Aneuploidy in human sperm: a review of the frequency and distribution of aneuploidy, effects of donor age and lifestyle factors. Cytogenet Cell Genet 90:219–226
13. Bispo AV, Dos Santos LO, Burégio-Frota P et al (2013) Effect of chromosome constitution variations on the expression of Turner phenotype. Genet Mol Res 12:4243–4250
14. Boyle B, Morris J, McConkey R et al (2014) Prevalence and risk of Down syndrome in monozygotic and dizygotic multiple pregnancies in Europe: implications for prenatal screening. BJOG. doi:10.1111/1471-0528.12574
15. Schwaibold EM, Bartels I, Küster H et al (2014) De novo duplication of chromosome 16p in a female infant with signs of neonatal hemochromatosis. Mol Cytogenet 7:7
16. Lamb NE, Yu K, Shaffer J et al (2005) Association between maternal age and meiotic recombination for trisomy 21. Am J Hum Genet 76:91–99
17. Cereda A, Carey JC (2012) The trisomy 18 syndrome. Orphanet J Rare Dis 7:81
18. Drugan A, Yaron Y, Zamir R et al (1999) Differential effect of advanced maternal age on prenatal diagnosis of trisomies 13, 18 and 21. Fetal Diagn Ther 14:181–184
19. De Souza E, Morris JK, EUROCAT Working Group (2010) Case-control analysis of paternal age and trisomic anomalies. Arch Dis Child 95:893–897
20. Wiener-Megnazi Z, Auslender R, Dirnfeld M (2012) Advanced paternal age and reproductive outcome. Asian J Androl 14:69–76
21. Yang Q, Wen SW, Leader A et al (2007) Paternal age and birth defects: how strong is the association? Hum Reprod 22:696–701
22. Chandirasekar R, Suresh K, Jayakumar R et al (2011) XRCC1 gene variants and possible links with chromosome aberrations and micronucleus in active and passive smokers. Environ Toxicol Pharmacol 32:185–192
23. Ladeira C, Viegas S, Carolino E et al (2013) The influence of genetic polymorphisms in XRCC3 and ADH5 genes on the frequency of genotoxicity biomarkers in workers exposed to formaldehyde. Environ Mol Mutagen 54:213–221
24. Jones KH, York TP, Juusola J et al (2011) Genetic and environmental influences on spontaneous micronuclei frequencies in children and adults: a twin study. Mutagenesis 26:745–752
25. Tan H, Wang Q, Wang A et al (2010) Influence of GSTs, CYP2E1 and mEH polymorphisms on 1, 3-butadiene-induced micronucleus frequency in Chinese workers. Toxicol Appl Pharmacol 247:198–203
26. Dada R, Thilagavathi J, Venkatesh S et al (2011) Genetic testing in male infertility. Open Reprod Sci J 3:42–56
27. Groth KA, Skakkebæk A, Høst C et al (2013) Clinical review: Klinefelter syndrome–a clinical update. J Clin Endocrinol Metab 98:20–30
28. Klinefelter HF, Reifenstein EC, Albright F (1942) Syndrome characterized by gynecomastia, aspermatogenesis without a-Leydigism, and increased excretion of follicle-stimulating hormone. J Clin Endocrinol 2:615–627
29. Wattendorf DJ, Muenke M (2005) Klinefelter syndrome. Am Fam Physician 72:2259–2262

30. Hassold T, Abruzzo M, Adkins K et al (1996) Human aneuploidy: incidence, origin, and etiology. Environ Mol Mutagen 28:167–175
31. Lanfranco F, Kamischke A, Zitzmann M et al (2004) Klinefelter's syndrome. Lancet 364:273–283
32. Smyth CM, Bremner WJ (1998) Klinefelter syndrome. Arch Intern Med 158:1309–1314
33. Georgiou I, Syrrou M, Pardalidis N et al (2006) Genetic and epigenetic risks of intracytoplasmic sperm injection method. Asian J Androl 8:643–673
34. Paduch DA, Fine RG, Bolyakov A et al (2008) New concepts in Klinefelter syndrome. Curr Opin Urol 18:621–627
35. Swerdlow AJ, Higgins CD, Schoemaker MJ et al (2005) Mortality in patients with Klinefelter syndrome in Britain: a cohort study. J Clin Endocrinol Metab 90:6516–6522
36. Bojesen A, Juul S, Birkebaek N et al (2004) Increased mortality in Klinefelter syndrome. J Clin Endocrinol Metab 89:3830–3834
37. Schiff JD, Palermo GD, Veeck LL et al (2005) Success of testicular sperm extraction [corrected] and intracytoplasmic sperm injection in men with Klinefelter syndrome. J Clin Endocrinol Metab 90:6263–6267
38. Komori S, Horiuchi I, Hamada Y et al (2004) Birth of healthy neonates after intracytoplasmic injection of ejaculated or testicular spermatozoa from men with nonmosaic Klinefelter's syndrome: a report of 2 cases. J Reprod Med 49:126–130
39. Ron-El R, Strassburger D, Gelman-Kohan S et al (2000) A 47, XXY fetus conceived after ICSI of spermatozoa from a patient with non-mosaic Klinefelter's syndrome: case report. Hum Reprod 15(8):1804–1806
40. Rogol AD, Tartaglia N (2010) Considerations for androgen therapy in children and adolescents with Klinefelter syndrome (47, XXY). Pediatr Endocrinol Rev 8(Suppl 1):145–150
41. Tempest HG, Simpson JL (2010) Role of preimplantation genetic diagnosis (PGD) in current infertility practice. Int J Infertil Fetal Med 1:1–10
42. Estop AM, Van Kirk V, Cieply K (1995) Segregation analysis of four translocations, t(2;18), t(3;15), t(5;7), and t(10;12), by sperm chromosome studies and a review of the literature. Cytogenet Cell Genet 70:80–87
43. Martin RH, Spriggs EL (1995) Sperm chromosome complements in a man heterozygous for a reciprocal translocation 46, XY, t(9;13) (q21.1;q21.2) and a review of the literature. Clin Genet 47:42–46
44. Alves C, Carvalho F, Cremades N et al (2002) Unique (Y;13) translocation in a male with oligozoospermia: cytogenetic and molecular studies. Eur J Hum Genet 10:467–474
45. Samli H, Samli MM, Solak M et al (2006) Genetic anomalies detected in patients with non-obstructive azoospermia and oligozoospermia. Arch Androl 52:263–267
46. Nagvenkar P, Desai K, Hinduja I et al (2005) Chromosomal studies in infertile men with oligozoospermia & non-obstructive azoospermia. Indian J Med Res 122:34–42
47. Gunel M, Cavkaytar S, Ceylaner G et al (2008) Azoospermia and cryptorchidism in a male with a de novo reciprocal t(Y;16) translocation. Genet Couns 19:277–280
48. Pabst B, Glaubitz R, Schalk T et al (2002) Reciprocal translocation between Y chromosome long arm euchromatin and the short arm of chromosome 1. Ann Genet 45:5–8
49. Therman E, Susman B, Denniston C (1989) The nonrandom participation of human acrocentric chromosomes in Robertsonian translocations. Ann Hum Genet 53(Pt 1):49–65
50. Ferlin A, Arredi B, Foresta C (2006) Genetic causes of male infertility. Reprod Toxicol 22:133–141
51. Dong Y, Du RC, Jiang YT et al (2012) Impact of chromosomal translocations on male infertility, semen quality, testicular volume and reproductive hormone levels. J Int Med Res 40: 2274–2283
52. Meschede D, Lemcke B, Exeler JR et al (1998) Chromosome abnormalities in 447 couples undergoing intracytoplasmic sperm injection-prevalence, types, sex distribution and reproductive relevance. Hum Reprod 13:576–582
53. Giraud F, Mattei JF (1975) Epidemiological aspects of trisomy 21. J Genet Hum 23(Suppl): 1–30

54. Briton-Jones C, Haines CJ (2000) Microdeletions on the long arm of the Y chromosome and their association with male-factor infertility. Hong Kong Med J 6:184–189
55. Kleiman SE, Yogev L, Gamzu R et al (1999) Genetic evaluation of infertile men. Hum Reprod 14:33–38
56. Navarro-Costa P, Goncalves J, Plancha CE (2010) The AZFc region of the Y chromosome: at the crossroads between genetic diversity and male infertility. Hum Reprod Update 16:525–542
57. Krausz C, Quintana-Murci L, McElreavey K (2000) Prognostic value of Y deletion analysis: what is the clinical prognostic value of Y chromosome microdeletion analysis? Hum Reprod 15:1431–1434
58. Dada R, Gupta NP, Kucheria K (2004) Yq microdeletions—azoospermia factor candidate genes and spermatogenic arrest. J Biomol Tech 15:176–183
59. Simoni M, Bakker E, Eurlings MC et al (1999) Laboratory guidelines for molecular diagnosis of Y-chromosomal microdeletions. Int J Androl 22(5):292–299
60. Kamp C, Huellen K, Fernandes S et al (2001) High deletion frequency of the complete AZFa sequence in men with Sertoli-cell-only syndrome. Mol Hum Reprod 7:987–994
61. Krausz C, Forti G, McElreavey K (2003) The Y chromosome and male fertility and infertility. Int J Androl 26:70–75
62. Tiepolo L, Zuffardi O (1976) Localization of factors controlling spermatogenesis in the non-fluorescent portion of the human Y chromosome long arm. Hum Genet 34:119–124
63. Vogt PH (2005) Azoospermia factor (AZF) in Yq11: towards a molecular understanding of its function for human male fertility and spermatogenesis. Reprod Biomed Online 10:81–93
64. Ma K, Mallidis C, Bhasin S (2000) The role of Y chromosome deletions in male infertility. Eur J Endocrinol 142:418–430
65. McLachlan RI, O'Bryan MK (2010) Clinical review: state of the art for genetic testing of infertile men. J Clin Endocrinol Metab 95:1013–1024
66. Pina-Neto JM, Carrara RC, Bisinella R et al (2006) Somatic cytogenetic and azoospermia factor gene microdeletion studies in infertile men. Braz J Med Biol Res 39:555–561
67. Massart A, Lissens W, Tournaye H et al (2012) Genetic causes of spermatogenic failure. Asian J Androl 14:40–48
68. Zhang F, Li L, Wang L et al (2013) Clinical characteristics and treatment of azoospermia and severe oligospermia patients with Y-chromosome microdeletions. Mol Reprod Dev 80:908–915
69. Harton GL, Tempest HG (2012) Chromosomal disorders and male infertility. Asian J Androl 14:32–39
70. Siffroi JP, Le Bourhis C, Krausz C et al (2000) Sex chromosome mosaicism in males carrying Y chromosome long arm deletions. Hum Reprod 15:2559–2562
71. Jaruzelska J, Korcz A, Wojda A et al (2001) Mosaicism for 45, X cell line may accentuate the severity of spermatogenic defects in men with AZFc deletion. J Med Genet 38:798–802
72. Brandell RA, Meilnik A, Liotta D et al (1998) AZFb deletions predict the absence of spermatozoa with testicular sperm extraction: preliminary report of a prognostic genetic test. Hum Reprod 13:2812–2815
73. Zhou-Cun A, Yang Y, Zhang SZ et al (2006) Chromosomal abnormality and Y chromosome microdeletion in Chinese patients with azoospermia or severe oligozoospermia. Yi Chuan Xue Bao 33:111–116
74. Jungwirth A, Giwercman A, Tournaye H et al; European Association of Urology Working Group on Male Infertility (2012) European Association of Urology guidelines on Male Infertility: the 2012 update. Eur Urol 62:324–332
75. Krausz C, Degl'Innocenti S (2006) Y chromosome and male infertility: update, 2006. Front Biosci 11:3049–3061
76. Simoni M, Bakker E, Eurlings MC et al (1999) Laboratory guidelines for molecular diagnosis of Y-chromosomal microdeletions. Int J Androl 22:292–299
77. Krausz C, Hoefsloot L, Simoni M et al (2014) EAA/EMQN best practice guidelines for molecular diagnosis of Y-chromosomal microdeletions: state-of-the-art 2013. Andrology 2: 5–19

78. Bienvenu T, Adjiman M, Thiounn N et al (1997) Molecular diagnosis of congenital bilateral absence of the vas deferens: analyses of the CFTR gene in 64 French patients. Ann Genet 40:5–9
79. Shah K, Sivapalan G, Gibbons N et al (2003) The genetic basis of infertility. Reproduction 126:13–25
80. Grangeia A, Niel F, Carvalho F et al (2004) Characterization of cystic fibrosis conductance transmembrane regulator gene mutations and IVS8 poly(T) variants in Portuguese patients with congenital absence of the vas deferens. Hum Reprod 19:2502–2508
81. Rommens JM, Iannuzzi MC, Kerem B et al (1989) Identification of the cystic fibrosis gene: chromosome walking and jumping. Science 245:1059–1065
82. Carrell DT, De Jonge C, Lamb DJ (2006) The genetics of male infertility: a field of study whose time is now. Arch Androl 52:269–274
83. Welsh MJ, Ramsey BW, Accurso F et al (2001) Cystic fibrosis. In: Scriver CL, Beaudet AL, Sly WS, Valle D (eds) The metabolic basis of inherited disease. McGraw-Hill, New York, pp 3799–3876
84. Kaplan E, Shwachman H, Perlmutter AD, Rule A, Khaw KT, Holsclaw DS (1968) Reproductive failure in males with cystic fibrosis. N Engl J Med 279:65–69
85. Landing BH, Wells TR, Wang CI (1969) Abnormality of the epididymis and vas deferens in cystic fibrosis. Arch Pathol 88:569–580
86. Rosenstein BJ, Cutting GR (1998) The diagnosis of cystic fibrosis: a consensus statement. Cystic Fibrosis Foundation Consensus Panel. J Pediatr 132:589–595
87. Anguiano A, Oates RD, Amos JA et al (1992) Congenital bilateral absence of the vas deferens. A primarily genital form of cystic fibrosis. JAMA 267:1794–1797
88. Lissens W, Mercier B, Tournaye H et al (1996) Cystic fibrosis and infertility caused by congenital bilateral absence of the vas deferens and related clinical entities. Hum Reprod 11(Suppl 4):55–78; discussion 79–80
89. Chillon M, Casals T, Mercier B et al (1995) Mutations in the cystic fibrosis gene in patients with congenital absence of the vas deferens. N Engl J Med 332:1475–1480
90. Hamada AJ, Esteves SC, Agarwal A (2013) A comprehensive review of genetics and genetic testing in azoospermia. Clinics (Sao Paulo) 68(Suppl 1):39–60
91. Weiske WH, Sälzler N, Schroeder-Printzen I et al (2000) Clinical findings in congenital absence of the vasa deferentia. Andrologia 32:13–18
92. Kolettis PN, Sandlow JI (2002) Clinical and genetic features of patients with congenital unilateral absence of the vas deferens. Urology 60:1073–1076
93. McCallum T, Milunsky J, Munarriz R et al (2001) Unilateral renal agenesis associated with congenital bilateral absence of the vas deferens: phenotypic findings and genetic considerations. Hum Reprod 16:282–288
94. Prader A, Labhart A, Willi H (1956) Ein Syndrom von Adipositas, Kleinwuchs, Kryptorchismus und Oligophrenic nach Myatonicartigem Zustand im Neugeborenalter. Schweiz Med Wochenschr 86:1260–1261
95. Cassidy SB (1997) Prader-Willi syndrome. J Med Genet 34:917–923
96. Vogels A, Van Den Ende J, Keymolen K et al (2004) Minimum prevalence, birth incidence and cause of death for Prader-Willi syndrome in Flanders. Eur J Hum Genet 12:238–240
97. Thomson AK, Glasson EJ, Bittles AH (2006) A long-term population-based clinical and morbidity review of Prader-Willi syndrome in Western Australia. J Intellect Disabil Res 50:69–78
98. Whittington JE, Holland AJ, Webb T et al (2001) Population prevalence and estimated birth incidence and mortality rate for people with Prader-Willi syndrome in one U.K. Health Region. J Med Genet 38:792–798
99. Nicholls RD, Knepper JL (2001) Genome organization, function, and imprinting in Prader-Willi and Angelman syndromes. Annu Rev Genomics Hum Genet 2:153–175
100. Cataletto M, Angulo M, Hertz G et al (2011) Prader-Willi syndrome: a primer for clinicians. Int J Pediatr Endocrinol 2011:12. doi:10.1186/1687-9856-2011-12

101. Goldstone AP, Holland AJ, Hauffa BP et al; speakers contributors at the Second Expert Meeting of the Comprehensive Care of Patients with PWS (2008) Recommendations for the diagnosis and management of Prader-Willi syndrome. J Clin Endocrinol Metab 93:4183–4197
102. Cassidy SB, Driscoll DJ (2009) Prader-Willi syndrome. Eur J Hum Genet 17:3–13
103. Crinò A, Schiaffini R, Ciampalini P et al (2003) Genetic obesity study group of Italian society of pediatric endocrinology and diabetology (SIEDP) Hypogonadism and pubertal development in Prader-Willi syndrome. Eur J Pediatr 162:327–333
104. Burman P, Ritzén EM, Lindgren AC (2001) Endocrine dysfunction in Prader-Willi syndrome: a review with special reference to GH. Endocr Rev 22:787–799
105. McCandless SE (2011) Clinical report health supervision for children with Prader-Willi syndrome. Pediatrics 127:195–204
106. Whittington JE, Butler JV, Holland AJ (2008) Pre-, peri- and postnatal complications in Prader-Willi syndrome in a U.K. sample. Early Hum Dev 84:331–336
107. Clayton-Smith J, Pembrey ME (1992) Angelman syndrome. J Med Genet 29:412–415
108. Steffenburg S, Gillberg CL, Steffenburg U et al (1996) Autism in Angelman syndrome: a population-based study. Pediatr Neurol 14:131–136
109. Petersen MB, Brondum-Nielsen K, Hansen LK et al (1995) Clinical, cytogenetic, and molecular diagnosis of Angelman syndrome: estimated prevalence rate in a Danish county. Am J Med Genet 60:261–262
110. Lossie AC, Driscoll DJ (1999) Transmission of Angelman syndrome by an affected mother. Genet Med 1:262–266
111. Williams CA, Driscoll DJ, Dagli AI (2010) Clinical and genetic aspects of Angelman syndrome. Genet Med 12:385–395

Male Idiopathic (Oligo) ± (Astheno) ± (Terato)-Spermia

9

Giorgio Cavallini

9.1 Definition

Male idiopathic (oligo)±(astheno)±(terato)-spermia (iOAT) is defined as a defective spermatogenesis of obscure etiology and is regarded as undetectable using common laboratory methods [1]. iOAT can be classified from a clinical point of view as isolated astheno±teratospermia (no alteration in sperm concentration), moderate iOAT (sperm concentration $<20 \times 10^6$/mL), or severe iOAT (sperm concentration $<5 \times 10^6$/mL) [2].

9.2 Epidemiology

iOAT affects approximately 30 % of infertile men and is one of the most common causes of infertility [1]. It is likely that its prevalence is increasing, in association with the progressive declining sperm count in men today [3].

9.3 Etiology

Descriptions of reputed causes of iOAT have at least two biases. Two patterns whose alterations are linked to male infertility with normal sperm parameters have been described: DNA damage and alterations of polymerase mitochondrial gamma gene (*POLG*) [4–6] (see Chap. 10). The sum of the percentages of patients with different causes of iOAT gave a result much higher than 100 %. This finding implies that the causes overlap, that the primary cause (if any) of iOAT is still unknown, and/or that more than one cause is needed to affect sperm patterns. The most likely hypothesis

G. Cavallini
Andrological Section, Gynepro-Medical Team, via Tranquillo Cremona 8,
Bologna 40137, Italy
e-mail: giorgiocavallini@libero.it

© Springer International Publishing Switzerland 2015
G. Cavallini, G. Beretta (eds.), *Clinical Management of Male Infertility*,
DOI 10.1007/978-3-319-08503-6_9

is the first; it has been demonstrated that iOAT sufferers comprise at least two different populations of infertile men [7].

9.3.1 Age

There is evidence that sperm motility declines progressively after age 30 years, although there is less evidence that a similar decline in sperm volume and concentration may also occur in typical presentations [8, 9].

9.3.2 Noninflammatory Functional Alteration in Post-testicular Organs

Low seminal concentration of prostate-specific antigen, zinc, fructose, and prostatic acid phosphatase [10], and low seminal activity of neutral α-glycosidase are linked to isolated asthenospermia in addition to increased viscoelasticity [11] and osmolarity of seminal plasma [12]. Alterations of epididymal methylation of spermatogenesis-specific genes have been suspected to be involved in the etiology of iOAT [13, 14]. Demethylation is critical for gene transcription.

9.3.3 Infective Agents

Chlamydia trachomatis (CT) and adenovirus (AV) infections have been regarded as being associated with iOAT; however, proof regarding the role of asymptomatic CT and/or AV infection in infertility is inconclusive [15, 16].

9.3.4 Genetic Factors

Approximately 10 % of rat genomes are specifically linked to spermatogenesis, and about 200 genes are regarded as critical for germ cell development [17]; this means that several genes might be involved in iOAT etiology. To be considered a key factor for iOAT, a gene must display all of the following characteristics: (1) it should be specifically expressed in the germ cell line, (2) its altered expression should be associated with iOAT; and (3) it should have an essential role in spermatogenesis [18]. Despite this restriction, several genes have been identified as causes of iOAT [19, 20]. (Diaginic) heredity and de novo mutations are the theoretical causes of the bad gene expression [1].

9.3.5 Mitochondrial Alterations

In asthenospermia, both mitochondrial membrane potential [21, 22] and DNA mitochondrial content [23, 24] are impaired.

9.3.6 Subtle Hormonal Alterations

A decreased luteinizing hormone (LH) pulse frequency has been found to occur in iOAT men whose amplitude parallels the severity of the disorder [25].

Molecular variants of LH have been associated with iOAT [26].

IOAT displays a shift toward lower testosterone (T) serum levels, lower calculated T index, and lower T/LH ratio, and a shift toward higher serum LH levels, higher 17-β2-estradiol (E2), and higher E2/T levels [27]. Increased E2 levels are postulated to contribute to the central suppression of gonadotropin production which, in turn, may decrease both T production and spermatogenesis [28]. E2 is derived mainly from the intratesticular and peripheral aromatization of androstenedione and T by aromatase, a product of the CYP19 gene. CYP 19A1 is a single-copy gene located on chromosome15q21.2. Aromatase polymorphisms have been shown to affect various estrogen-dependent diseases in men and women. The most commonly studied aromatase polymorphism is the tetranucleotide Tyrosine-Tyrosine-Tyrosine-Adenine [TTTA] repeat polymorphism [TTTAn] present in intron 4 of the CYP 19A1 gene. This polymorphism is associated with the activity of the aromatase enzyme both in vivo and in vitro [29]. Higher numbers of TTTA repeats (>7 repeats) in the aromatase gene are associated with a negative relationship between obesity and sperm count. The effect of obesity on E2 and sperm count appears to be absent in men with fewer (≤7) repeats [30].

9.3.7 Environmental Pollutants

Environmental pollutants are regarded as capable of deteriorating semen quality. Chapter 16 is specifically dedicated to this aspect.

9.4 Pathogenesis

The aforementioned causes affect spermatogenesis. Impaired spermatogenesis leads to increased reactive oxygen species (ROS) and unbalanced germ cell apoptosis.

9.4.1 Increased ROS

ROS originate from the cellular physiologic metabolism of O_2 in aerobic conditions, and are mainly produced by leukocytes and immature gametes. Immature gametes are common findings in iOAT. ROS are short-lived chemical intermediates containing one or more electrons with unpaired spins. All spermatozoa structures can be attacked and denatured by ROS [1, 31], ultimately resulting in death and/or irreversible damage. Physiologic (low) levels of ROS exert critical function in normal sperm physiology, such as fertilizing ability (acrosome reaction, hyperactivation, capacitation, and chemotaxis) and sperm motility; whereas increased ROS generation and/or decreased antioxidant capacity leads to the imbalance between oxidation and reduction in living systems, which is called sperm oxidative stress. This condition was widely considered to be a significant contributory factor to sperm DNA damage/apoptosis, lipid peroxidation, and reduced motility, which, in turn, increased the risk of male factor infertility/subfertility and birth defects [31].

9.4.2 Modified Apoptosis

Apoptosis (programmed cell death) is a physiologic mechanism aimed at achieving optimal Sertoli cell/gamete ratio and removing damaged gametes [32]. The range of stimuli that triggers this activity is impressively broad and includes various forms of electromagnetic radiation, environmental toxicants, heavy metals, and chemotherapeutic agents [33–37]. In addition, genetic perturbation of the germ cell line occurs through, for example, overexpression of SPATA17 [38] or androgen-binding protein [39], or deletion of key genes involved in the regulation of spermatogenesis [40–42]. The impression given is that if spermatogenesis is disrupted in any way, the germ cells tend to default to an apoptotic state. The stage of spermatogenesis when apoptosis is induced appears to be predominantly pachytene spermatocytes, and the Fas (fibroblast-associated death receptor)/Fas ligand and caspase systems seems to be the major mediators of this process [34].

9.5 Diagnosis

iOAT is commonly diagnosed by exclusion; the differential diagnosis is presented in Table 9.1.

Table 9.1 Differential diagnosis of male infertility [2]

Reproductive failure mechanism		Methods of diagnosis
Chromosomal	X chromosome disorders	Objective examination, Y microdeletion detection, karyotype screening of cystic fibrosis, hormonal profiles, androgen receptor detection, semen analysis
	Y chromosome disorders	
	Autosomal disorders	
Developmental	Hypospadias	Clinical history, objective examination, semen analysis, scrotal echography
	Ductal obstruction	
	Didymal-epididymal interruption	

Table 9.1 (continued)

Reproductive failure mechanism		Methods of diagnosis
Testicular pathology	Cryptorchidism	Clinical history, objective examination, semen analysis, scrotal echography
	Ectopic testicle	
	Retarded descent	
	(Floating testicle?)	
	Testicular tumors	
	Bilateral atrophy	
	Trauma	
	Testicular torsion	
Genital tract inflammation	Urethritis	Clinical history, objective examination, semen analysis, scrotal echography, urethral swab, urine analysis, sperm and urine cultural analysis
	Prostatitis	
	Epididymitis	
	Orchitis	
Varicocele		Objective examination, scrotal bilateral echo-color Doppler examination, semen analysis
Endocrine	Pituitary disorders	Hormonal profiles
	Hypothalamic disorders	Semen analysis
	Testicle disorders	
	Thyroid disorders	
	Adrenal gland disorders	
Iatrogenic	Surgery	Clinical history, objective examination, semen analysis
	Drugs	
	Radiation	
Sexually related causes	Erectile deficiency	Clinical history, semen analysis
	Disturbed ejaculation	
General diseases	Renal diseases	
	Liver diseases	
	Neurologic diseases	
	Gastrointestinal diseases	
	Hematologic diseases	
	Autoimmune diseases	
	Infectious diseases (AIDS)	
	Psoriasis	
	Sarcoidosis	
	Diabetes	
Idiopathic oligoasthenoteratospermia		Semen analysis, exclusion criteria

9.6 Therapy

Therapy for iOAT is commonly regarded as empiric, because it is not possible in the current outpatient clinical setting to define the exact etiology of the spermatogenetic disorder of each iOAT patient. A number of therapies have been proposed, the most effective of which, according to author's experience and literature review, are reported here. Obviously these therapies might improve the sperm count in the majority of patients but not in all, and these therapies should be intended as symptomatic therapies: i.e., sperm count is improved as long as these therapies are administered, and decrease immediately after their suspension. Therapies should be administered for at least 3 months, because a stem cell requires about 61 days to achieve the final status of mature spermatozoon [43]. A rough therapeutic classification can be compiled on the basis of sperm analysis results.

9.6.1 Isolated (Astheno) ± (Terato)-Spermia

Coenzyme Q10 100 mg twice daily for at least 3 months. Coenzyme Q10 is a lipophilic antioxidant agent and should be administered after meals. Galenic preparations should use lipophilic excipients (e.g., cocoa butter) [44].

9.6.2 Oligo-Astheno-Teratospermia with Sperm Concentration >5 × 10⁶/mL

l-*Carnitine* 1 g twice daily; *acetyl*-l-*carnitine* 500 mg twice daily; *cinnoxicam* 30 mg, one tablet every 4 days after the main meal. These drugs are antioxidant agents [45, 46].

9.6.3 All Degrees of Dyspermia with Serum Follicle-Stimulating Hormone <2 mIU/mL

Intramuscular *recombinant Follicle-Stimulating Hormone (FSH)* 100–300 IU every 2 days. FSH stimulates Sertoli cell function and spermatogenesis [47, 48].

9.6.4 All Degrees of Dyspermia with a low (<10) T/E2 Ratio

These dyspermias have exhibited an increased sperm count after *letrozole* (2.5 mg/day) and/or *anastrozole* (1 mg/day) treatment. Nonobstructive azoospermic patients with T/E2 ratio <10 also had their sperm count increased with letrozole and/or anastrozole treatment. Letrozole and anastrozole are members of a novel class of nonsteroidal, hormone-targeting agents used for breast cancer therapy. They reversibly inhibit the aromatase enzyme, which converts the androgen precursors in adipose tissue to E2. Blocking of estrogen production has been shown to provoke increased gonadotropin and androgen levels in the blood and a parallel E2 decrease, resulting in spermatogenesis stimulation [49, 50].

9.7 Prognosis

Prognosis is difficult to define in these patients, mainly because of the empiric nature of the therapies. However, antioxidant drugs and aromatase inhibitors significantly lower the number of couples that might require treatment with assisted reproduction to achieve a pregnancy [51].

References

1. Cavallini G (2006) Male idiopathic oligoasthenoteratospermia. Asian J Androl 8:143–157
2. World Health Organization (2010) WHO manual for the examination and processing of human semen, 5th edn. Cambridge University Press, Cambridge
3. Burton A (2013) Study suggests long-term decline in French sperm quality. Environ Health Perspect 121:46–47
4. Saleh RA, Agarwal A, Nelson DR, Nada EA, El-Tonsy MH, Alvarez JG, Thomas AJ Jr, Sharma RK (2002) Increased sperm nuclear DNA damage in normozoospermic infertile men: a prospective study. Fertil Steril 78:313–318
5. Jensen M, Leffers H, Petersen JH, Nyboe Andersen A, Jørgensen N, Carlsen E, Jensen TK, Skakkebaek NE, Rajpert-De Meyts E (2004) Frequent polymorphism of the mitochondrial DNA polymerase gamma gene [POLG] in patients with normal spermiograms and unexplained subfertility. Hum Reprod 19:65–70
6. Esteves SC (2013) A clinical appraisal of the genetic basis in unexplained male infertility. J Hum Reprod Sci 6:176–182
7. Cavallini G, Crippa A, Magli MC, Cavallini N, Ferraretti AP, Gianaroli L (2008) A study to sustain the hypothesis of the multiple genesis of oligoasthenoteratospermia in human idiopathic infertile males. Biol Reprod 79:667–673
8. Kidd SA, Eskenazi B, Wyrobek AJ (2001) Effects of male age on semen quality and fertility: a review of the literature. Fertil Steril 75:237–248
9. Zhu QX, Meads C, Lu ML, Wu JQ, Zhou WJ, Gao ES (2011) Turning point of age for semen quality: a population-based study in Chinese men. Fertil Steril 96:572–576
10. Carpino A, Sisci D, Aquila S, Salerno M, Siciliano L, Sessa M, Andò S (1994) Adnexal gland secretion markers in unexplained asthenozoospermia. Arch Androl 32:37–43
11. ELzanaty S, Malm J, Giwercman A (2004) Visco-elasticity of seminal fluid in relation to the epididymal and accessory sex gland function and its impact on sperm motility. Int J Androl 27:94–100
12. Rossato M, Balercia G, Lucarelli G, Foresta C, Mantero F (2002) Role of seminal osmolarity in the reduction of human sperm motility. Int J Androl 25:230–235
13. Ariel M, Robinson E, McCarrey JR, Cedar H (1995) Gamete-specific methylation correlates with imprinting of the murine Xist gene. Nat Genet 9:312–315
14. Rotondo JC, Selvatici R, Di Domenico M, Marci R, Vesce F, Tognon M, Martini F (2013) Methylation loss at H19 imprinted gene correlates with methylenetetrahydrofolate reductase gene promoter hypermethylation in semen samples from infertile males. Epigenetics 8:990–997
15. Eggert-Kruse W, Rohr G, Demirakca T, Rusu R, Näher H, Petzoldt D, Runnebaum B (1997) Chlamydial serology in 1303 asymptomatic subfertile couples. Hum Reprod 12:1464–1475

16. Schlehofer JR, Boeke C, Reuland M, Eggert-Kruse W (2012) Presence of DNA of adeno-associated virus in subfertile couples, but no association with fertility factors. Hum Reprod 27:770–778
17. Schlecht U, Demougin P, Koch R, Hermida L, Wiederkehr C, Descombes P, Pineau C, Jégou B, Primig M (2004) Expression profiling of mammalian male meiosis and gametogenesis identifies novel candidate genes for roles in the regulation of fertility. Mol Biol Cell 15:1031–1043
18. Mäkelä S, Eklund R, Lähdetie J, Mikkola M, Hovatta O, Kere J (2005) Mutational analysis of the human SLC26A8 gene: exclusion as a candidate for male infertility due to primary spermatogenic failure. Mol Hum Reprod 11:129–132
19. O'Flynn O'Brien KL, Varghese AC, Agarwal A (2010) The genetic causes of male factor infertility: a review. Fertil Steril 93:1–12
20. Ferlin A, Raicu F, Gatta V, Zuccarello D, Palka G, Foresta C (2007) Male infertility: role of genetic background. Reprod Biomed Online 14:734–745
21. Kasai T, Ogawa K, Mizuno K, Nagai S, Uchida Y, Ohta S, Fujie M, Suzuki K, Hirata S, Hoshi K (2002) Relationship between sperm mitochondrial membrane potential, sperm motility, and fertility potential. Asian J Androl 4:97–103
22. Marchetti C, Jouy N, Leroy-Martin B, Defossez A, Formstecher P, Marchetti P (2004) Comparison of four fluorochromes for the detection of the inner mitochondrial membrane potential in human spermatozoa and their correlation with sperm motility. Hum Reprod 19:2267–2276
23. Kao SH, Chao HT, Liu HW, Liao TL, Wei YH (2004) Sperm mitochondrial DNA depletion in men with asthenospermia. Fertil Steril 82:66–73
24. Song GJ, Lewis V (2008) Mitochondrial DNA integrity and copy number in sperm from infertile men. Fertil Steril 90:2238–2244
25. Odabas O, Atilla MK, Yilmaz Y, Sekeroglu MR, Sengul E, Aydin S (2002) Luteinizing hormone pulse frequency and amplitude in azoospermic, oligozoospermic and normal fertile men in Turkey. Asian J Androl 4:156–158
26. Ramanujam LN, Liao WX, Roy AC, Ng SC (2000) Association of molecular variants of luteinizing hormone with male infertility. Hum Reprod 15:925–928
27. Andersson AM, Jørgensen N, Frydelund-Larsen L, Rajpert-De Meyts E, Skakkebaek NE (2004) Impaired Leydig cell function in infertile men: a study of 357 idiopathic infertile men and 318 proven fertile controls. J Clin Endocrinol Metab 89:3161–3167
28. Zhang Q, Bai Q, Yuan Y, Liu P, Qiao J (2010) Assessment of seminal estradiol and testosterone levels as predictors of human spermatogenesis. J Androl 31:215–220
29. Gennari L, Masi L, Merlotti D, Picariello L, Falchetti A (2004) A polymorphic CYP19 TTTA repeat influences aromatase activity and estrogen levels in elderly men: effects on bone metabolism. J Clin Endocrinol Metab 89:2803–2810
30. Hammoud AO, Griffin J, Meikle AW, Gibson M, Peterson CM (2010) Association of aromatase [TTTAn] repeat polymorphism length and the relationship between obesity and decreased sperm concentration. Hum Reprod 25:3146–3151
31. Chen SJ, Allam JP, Duan YG, Haidl G (2013) Influence of reactive oxygen species on human sperm functions and fertilizing capacity including therapeutical approaches. Arch Gynecol Obstet 288:191–199
32. Aitken RJ, Baker MA (2013) Causes and consequences of apoptosis in spermatozoa; contributions to infertility and impacts on development. Int J Dev Biol 57:265–272
33. Alam MS, Ohsako S, Tay TW, Tsunekawa N, Kanai Y, Kurohmaru M (2010) Di[n-butyl] phthalate induces vimentin filaments disruption in rat Sertoli cells: a possible relation with spermatogenic cell apoptosis. Anat Histol Embryol 39:186–193
34. Li YJ, Song TB, Cai YY, Zhou JS, Song X, Zhao X, Wu XL (2009) Bisphenol A exposure induces apoptosis and upregulation of Fas/FasL and caspase-3 expression in the testes of mice. Toxicol Sci 108:427–436
35. Shaha C, Tripathi R, Mishra DP (2010) Male germ cell apoptosis: regulation and biology. Philos Trans R Soc Lond B Biol Sci 365:1501–1515

36. Wang C, Cui YG, Wang XH, Jia Y, Sinha Hikim A, Lue YH, Tong JS, Qian LX, Sha JH, Zhou ZM, Hull L, Leung A, Swerdloff RS (2007) Transient scrotal hyperthermia and levonorgestrel enhance testosterone-induced spermatogenesis suppression in men through increased germ cell apoptosis. J Clin Endocrinol Metab 92:3292–3304
37. Xu G, Zhou G, Jin T, Zhou T, Hammarström S, Bergh A, Nordberg G (1999) Apoptosis and p53 gene expression in male reproductive tissues of cadmium exposed rats. Biometals 12:131–139
38. Nie DS, Liu Y, Juan H, Yang X (2013) Overexpression of human SPATA17 protein induces germ cell apoptosis in transgenic male mice. Mol Biol Rep 40:1905–1910
39. Jeyaraj DA, Grossman G, Petrusz P (2003) Dynamics of testicular germ cell apoptosis in normal mice and transgenic mice overexpressing rat androgen-binding protein. Reprod Biol Endocrinol 12:48–49
40. Gutti RK, Tsai-Morris CH, Dufau ML (2008) Gonadotropin-regulated testicular helicase [DDX25], an essential regulator of spermatogenesis, prevents testicular germ cell apoptosis. J Biol Chem 283:17055–17064
41. Kosir R, Juvan P, Perse M, Budefeld T, Majdic G, Fink M, Sassone-Corsi P, Rozman D (2012) Novel insights into the downstream pathways and targets controlled by transcription factors CREM in the testis. PLoS One 7(2):e31798. doi:10.1371/journal.pone.0031798
42. Liu Z, Zhou S, Liao L, Chen X, Meistrich M, Xu J (2010) Jmjd1a demethylase-regulated histone modification is essential for cAMP-response element modulator-regulated gene expression and spermatogenesis. J Biol Chem 285:2758–2770
43. Anawalt BD (2013) Approach to male infertility and induction of spermatogenesis. J Clin Endocrinol Metab 98:3532–3542
44. Safarinejad MR, Safarinejad S, Shafiei N, Safarinejad S (2012) Effects of the reduced form of coenzyme Q10 (ubiquinol) on semen parameters in men with idiopathic infertility: a double-blind, placebo controlled, randomized study. J Urol 188:526–531
45. Cavallini G, Ferraretti AP, Gianaroli L, Biagiotti G, Vitali G (2004) Cinnoxicam and L-carnitine/acetyl-L-carnitine treatment for idiopathic and varicocele-associated oligoasthenospermia. J Androl 25:761–770
46. Cavallini G, Magli MC, Crippa A, Ferraretti AP, Gianaroli L (2012) Reduction in sperm aneuploidy levels in severe oligoasthenoteratospermic patients after medical therapy: a preliminary report. Asian J Androl 14:591–598
47. Foresta C, Bettella A, Merico M, Garolla A, Ferlin A, Rossato M (2002) Use of recombinant human follicle-stimulating hormone in the treatment of male factor infertility. Fertil Steril 77(2):238–244
48. Paradisi R, Natali F, Fabbri R, Battaglia C, Seracchioli R, Venturoli S (2013) Evidence for a stimulatory role of high doses of recombinant human follicle-stimulating hormone in the treatment of male-factor infertility. Andrologia. doi:10.1111/and.12194. [Epub ahead of print]
49. Schlegel PN (2012) Aromatase inhibitors for male infertility. Fertil Steril 98:1359–1362
50. Cavallini G, Biagiotti G, Bolzon E (2013) Multivariate analysis to predict letrozole efficacy in improving sperm count of non-obstructive azoospermic and cryptozoospermic patients: a pilot study. Asian J Androl 15:806–811
51. Comhaire F, Decleer W (2012) Comparing the effectiveness of infertility treatments by numbers needed to treat (NNT). Andrologia 44:401–404

Obesity and Male Infertility

10

Carlo Maretti

10.1 Definition

Infertility means not being able to get pregnant after a year of constant and unprotected intercourses [1]. Infertility and sterility are two very different concepts. Sterility is the permanent inability to reproduce. Infertility, on the other hand, can be either a permanent or temporary inability for fertilization to occur, because of one or more interfering factors [1]. In recent decades, the quality of the male semen compared to the 1999 classification by the World Health Organization (WHO) has become increasingly worse so that in 2010 (Table 10.1) normospermia was defined as having a sperm concentration ≥15 mil/ml, a progressive motility ≥32 %, and a morphology with a percentage of normal forms ≥4 % where for each parameter the percentile was identified, and where the minimum parameter corresponded to the 5th percentile, which meant that out of 100 people, 95 % had the best fertility parameters. In other words, just referring to the morphology, only 5 % of people had 4 % of fertile sperm in their normal form [2].

Obesity, defined as abnormal or excessive fat accumulation that presents a risk to health, has important effects on fertility [3].

Obesity is a multifactorial disease caused by energy imbalance between calories consumed and calories expended, resulting in the accumulation of body fat. The condition of obesity is defined using the body mass index (BMI) which is a biometric datum, expressed as the ratio between the individual's weight and the square of the height, and it is used as an indicator of ideal weight (Table 10.2) [4].

C. Maretti
Department of Andrology, Centro Medico CIRM, Via Somaglia 10, Piacenza 29121, Italy
e-mail: andrologia@tin.it

Table 10.1 Spermiogram parameters by the WHO [2]

Spermiogram parameters by the World Health Organization	1999 ed.	2010 ed.
Volume	≥ 2 ml	≥ 1.5 ml
Concentration	20 mil/ml	15 mil/ml
Ntot sperm cells	40 mil	39 mil
Total motility	≥ 50 %	≥ 40 %
Progressive motility	≥ 25 %	≥ 32 %
Morphology % normal	≥ 30 %	≥ 4 %
Vitality	≥ 50 %	≥ 58 %

Table 10.2 The worldwide classification of the body mass index (BMI) [4]

	BMI (kg/m^2)	
Classification	Main cutoff points	Additional cutoff points
Underweight	<18.50	<18.50
Critical thinness	<16.00	<16.00
Moderate thinness	16.00–16.99	16.00–16.99
Mild thinness	17.00–18.49	17.00–18.49
Normal weight	18.50–24.99	18.50–22.99
		23.00–24.99
Overweight	≥ 25.00	≥ 25.00
Pre-obese	25.00–29.99	25.00–27.49
		27.50–29.99
Obese	≥ 30.00	≥ 30.00
Obese class I	30.00–34.99	30.00–32.49
		32.50–34.99
Obese class II	35.00–39.99	35.00–37.49
		37.50–39.99
Obese class III	≥ 40.00	≥ 40.00

10.2 Epidemiology

Infertility is caused by male factors in 25.5 % of infertile couples [5]. Body mass index or BMI is a simple and widely used method for estimating body fat mass. The healthy BMI range varies with age and sex; obesity in children and adolescents is defined as a BMI greater than the 95th percentile. In children, obesity is more severe and shows an even distribution of the body fat mass, which involves the whole body, including the upper and lower limbs, normally excluded by the adult obesity which has a typical central arrangement. Obesity is one of the most common diseases among the industrialized countries where the incidence rates are increasing so much that according to the data of the WHO, 54 % of the adult population is overweight

Table 10.3 Causal factors of couple's infertility [5]

Causal factors of couple's infertility	(%)
Male factor	25.5
Ovulatory endocrine infertility	16.9
Endometriosis	6.0
Male or female factor	17.3
Unexplained infertility	29.1
Others	5.3

and 25 % is obese [4]. Infertility, especially in the highly industrialized countries, contributes to the dramatic fall in the birth rate. Epidemiological studies in the USA sorted out that the male fertility has been gradually reduced in the industrialized countries since 1936 by recording a severe incidence of obesity. Over the past 70 years, the semen quality got worse, with an incidence in the male population between 15 and 18 % [3] (Table 10.3).

Numerous data in the medical literature confirm that the reduction in male fertility depends on nutritional factors [6–8]. There is an inverse correlation between BMI and the main hormones that mediate male fertility, where the obese have increased levels of estrogen and low levels of FSH, LH, inhibin B, and total and free testosterone [9–11]. Several studies confirm that the increase in BMI would refer to a reduction in sperm concentration (oligospermia), motility, and sperm morphology (asthenoteratospermia) and to an increase in nemaspermic DNA fragmentation (Table 10.4) [23–25].

10.3 Etiopathology

There is a close relationship between fertility and lifestyles [26]. As a matter of fact, the reduction of fertility in men is also connected to nutritional factors [6]. Energy intake in obese subjects is chronically larger than the energy expenditure, but the phenomena that give rise to this chronic alteration are not known. However, in humans, we can clarify the physiopathological mechanisms that regulate energetic homeostasis through constant regulation of body weight and balance between body fat and lean mass [27].

It has been reported that overweight and obese men have an up to 50 % higher rate of subfertility when compared to normal-weight men [21]. This effect persists even when confounding factors such as diseases, age, smoking, alcohol use, and obese female partner have been controlled [3]. Obesity is strongly linked to reduced spermatogenesis, poor quality of sperm, and a reduced percentage of normal sperm morphology [23]. Men's diets, in particular the amount and type of different fats they eat, could be associated with their semen quality. According to the results of a study [14], it has been found that men who ate omega-3 polyunsaturated fats (the type of fat often found in fish and plant oils) had better-formed sperm than men who ate less. A diet full of saturated fatty acids would cause a reduction in sperm count, while a diet rich in omega-3 fatty acids would

Table 10.4 Scientific evidence between obesity and male infertility

Reports	Number of patients	People	Results/conclusion	Ratio BMI/infertility
Eisenberg et al. [12]	501	Couples from a longitudinal investigation on infertility and environment	No modified semen parameters No DNA fragmentation in the sperm cell	No
Jensen et al. [13]	701	Cross-sectional study of young men attending the military service	A high intake of saturated fats reduces the sperm concentration and total sperm count	Yes
Attaman et al. [14]	99	Men attending fertility clinic	A higher intake of omega-3 fats is positively related to sperm morphology	Yes
Fariello et al. [15]	305	Male patients of a cross-sectional study	Decreased progressive motility Increased sperm DNA fragmentation	Yes
Rybar et al. [16]	153	Men of infertile couples	No modified semen parameters	No
Martini et al. [17]	794	Male patients of a blind prospective study	Deleterious effects of obesity on seminal quality	Yes
Safarinejad [18]	160	Fertile and infertile men	A higher intake of omega-3 fats is positively related to semen parameters	Yes
Chavarro et al. [19]	483	Men of infertile couples	Hypospermia Reduction of sperm cell if BMI >35 DNA fragmentation in the sperm cell	Yes
Hofny et al. [20]	122	Only fertile and infertile obese men	Reduction in the sperm count and motility Increase of atypical sperm cells, sexual hormones alteration	Yes
Pauli et al. [21]	87	BMI 16.1–7.0 kg/m^2	Any meaningless correlations with sperm parameters, reduced fertility	Yes/no
Agbaje et al. [22]	56	Men with diabetes type 2	DNA fragmentation and reduction of the semen volume	Yes

contribute to a better sperm morphology. Men with a high intake of saturated fat have a 35 % lower total sperm count than men with a low intake and a 38 % lower sperm concentration [13]. A number of previous studies had investigated the link between BMI and semen quality, with mixed results (Table 10.4). The mechanisms by which obesity is associated with hypogonadism are mostly unknown, but it is likely that insulin or other hormonal factors released from the adipose tissue may have a role in regulating the production of pituitary LH [22]. In men, one of the main causes of infertility determined by obesity is closely related to the hyperactivity of aromatase, an enzyme which is present in high percentage in the so-called white adipose tissue, which converts testosterone into estradiol. The increase of estradiol concentration is proportional to the quantity of adipose tissue, and estrogens exert a negative feedback action on the pituitary secretion of both FSH and LH, the essential hormones for the normal growth and differentiation of sperm [28]. The white adipose tissue is also the main site of synthesis of leptin, a hormone which regulates the energetic stability and body weight by modulating the energy intake and expenditure at the level of the central nervous system. So an increase in fat mass, resulting from a caloric excess, corresponds to an increased secretion of the hormone on behalf of the adipose tissue. Leptin circulates in plasma at concentrations that parallel the amount of fat reserves. In obese males, androgen levels decline in proportion to the degree of obesity. When leptin is produced in exaggerate amounts, it can reduce the level of androgens, and as its receptors are found in the testicular tissue, this can have a direct effect on the functionality of the sperm [20].

Another characteristic of the adipose tissue that may interfere on male fertility is the increased production of resistin, a protein associated with insulin resistance. Plasma levels of this cytokine are increased in obese individuals [29]. Hyperinsulinemia is related to inhibition of spermatogenesis, and it also produces a deterioration of spermatic DNA, which causes not only a reduction in fertility but also a higher incidence of spontaneous abortions in female partners [22].

Obesity and diabetes mellitus are insulin-resistant states with different abnormalities in oxidative stress, protein glycation, and cellular processes that lead to impaired endothelial function, vascular inflammation, and hemostasis: processes which give rise to impaired function of the microcirculation [22]. A large body of scientific evidences indicates that overweight or obese men frequently suffer from erectile dysfunction (ED) which is a cause of infertility. Sedentary life, prolonged sitting, and fat deposition in the lower abdomen can reduce male fertility, likely through increased testicular temperature to the level of body core temperature [30].

An excessive intake of metabolizable food, especially carbohydrates and fats, subdues the individual to an oxidative stress with negative echoes on the reproductive area. In a healthy body there is a balance between the oxidative mechanisms and the antioxidant defenses. In normal conditions, the toxic potential of free radicals (ROS) is neutralized by a complex system of antioxidant factors that represents our physiological mechanism of defense. The relationship between oxidant factors and antioxidant defenses is the so-called oxidative balance. Oxidative stress is, therefore, the expression of biological damage that occurs when the prooxidant factors (drugs, toxic substances, radiations, inflammations, etc.) exceed the endogenous antioxidant defenses (enzymes such as superoxide dismutase, coenzyme Q10, catalase, peroxidase, etc.) and the exogenous ones (antioxidants found in food). Obesity is a pathological condition which causes oxidative stress with increased ROS in sperm causing its decreased quality. During the last years, andrologists' interest on the diagnostics and treatment of male infertility has focused on the role of ROS in the pathogenesis of male infertility with harmful effects on sperm membrane rich in polyunsaturated fatty acids. The increased production of ROS and the related oxidative stress associated with obesity may be therefore responsible for the increased lipidic peroxidation damage to the sperm cell membrane [31, 32]. Not only the quantity but also the quality of food can have an effect on male fertility, and in recent years a lot of attention has been paid to the so-called endocrine-disrupting compounds, i.e., substances which have a structural similarity to the endogenous hormones, and therefore they are able to mime the hormones themselves, interacting with their transport proteins. A substantial number of environmental pollutants, such as polychlorinated biphenyls, dioxins, polycyclic aromatic hydrocarbons, phthalates, bisphenol A, alkylphenols, pesticides, and heavy metals (arsenic, cadmium, lead, mercury), have shown to interfere with endocrine function as they are released in the environment in different ways such as smoke, sewage, and careless use of pesticides with the direct release on the food. These substances can cause reproductive problems by reducing either the concentration of sperm or its quality [33].

10.4 Diagnosis and Therapy

In this context, prevention has been of great importance in order to protect and preserve the fertility of the individual since childhood. Smoking, obesity or excessive thinness, different environmental substances, physical inactivity, and even unrestrained physical activity are some of the major risk factors capable of influencing the sexual and reproductive health of an individual [34].

In the first 2 years of life, a hyperalimentation can cause not only a hypertrophy of fat cells but can lead to hyperplasia that will develop to a sure adult obesity [35]. The best treatment of male infertility is the correct diagnosis. The andrologist, through a careful diagnostic process, can identify which is the most appropriate medical and/or surgical treatment for the infertile patient and has an important role in referring eventually the infertile couple to medically assisted procreation. Obesity is often associated with metabolic alterations (diabetes, hypertension, dyslipidemia, hyperuricemia) that are important cardiovascular risk factors which may have an impact on male sexual and reproductive health and in determining psychological disorders. Therefore, in the diagnostic algorithm of morbid obesity, it is essential to weigh the patient, to examine some important parameters about his family history, to know his waist circumference and blood pressure, and to ask for a few diagnostic tests which are essential to a correct understanding of the problems [35]. Laboratory tests are of considerable importance to assess glucose tolerance and lipid and hormone profile as well as an assessment of the seminal fluid. In particular, it is necessary to evaluate the hypothalamic-pituitary-gonadal axis through the determination of FSH, LH, estradiol, and total testosterone and the examination of seminal fluid according to the WHO criteria of 2010 (Table 10.1) [17].

Once the patient's clinical history, state of health, behavior, and food habits have been pointed out, a therapeutic integrated path referring to the different pathologies will be started. Since obesity is an altered balance between energy consumption and caloric intake, dietary therapy and physical activity must become part of a rehabilitation program. Weight reduction (5–10 % of initial body weight) leads to benefits in terms of morbidity and mortality: it is shown that a lasting weight loss allows significant improvements of all the metabolic syndrome parameters, and in particular the reduction of visceral fat is associated with an improvement of the male reproductive function [35]. Moreover, a psychological evaluation is essential. Improving fertility can be a strong motivation for weight loss [36]. Dietary antioxidants may be beneficial in reducing sperm DNA damage, in infertile obese men [37].

In a male who suffers from obesity, diabetes, or metabolic syndrome, with a reduced fertility and hypogonadotropic hypogonadism, it is possible to evaluate a treatment with antiestrogens or aromatase inhibitors that, if properly prescribed, can improve the quantitative and qualitative characteristics of the seminal fluid. Antiestrogens have the ability to bind to estrogen receptors, both at the hypothalamic and the peripheral levels in a competitive manner, thus inducing an increase in plasma levels of gonadotropins and then of intratesticular testosterone [38]. The pharmacological effect on spermatogenesis should be manifested through increased concentrations of FSH, LH, and testosterone, although a direct effect on spermatogenesis cannot be excluded. The first used antiestrogen was clomiphene citrate, replaced by tamoxifen citrate in recent years [39]. Estradiol is derived from the conversion of testosterone, mediated by the aromatase system which occurs in the testicles and peripheral, especially in adipose, tissues. Testolactone, an inhibitor of aromatase, can improve the testicular function through two mechanisms: a decrease of the concentrations of estradiol and a stimulation of the secretion of gonadotropins from the pituitary through a block of the inhibitory feedback exerted by estradiol. Anastrozole, a selective inhibitor of aromatase, at a dose of 1 mg per day, and letrozole (2.5 mg/day) seem to be comparable to the testolactone for its effects on spermatogenesis [28].

The use of these molecules is interesting especially in patients with an altered testosterone/estradiol ratio, as occurs in obese subjects. Further studies will be necessary to evaluate the effectiveness of these drugs in the treatment of male infertility in the obese because of the small number of studied subjects.

References

1. Stephen EH, Chandra A (2006) Declining estimates of infertility in the United States: 1982–2002. Fertil Steril 86(3):516–523
2. World Health Organization (2010) WHO laboratory manual for the examination and processing of human semen, 5th edn. WHO Press, Geneva
3. Sallmén M, Sandler DP, Hoppin JA, Blair A, Baird DD (2006) Reduced fertility among overweight and obese men. Epidemiology 17(5):520–523
4. World Health Organization (1998) Obesity: preventing and managing the global epidemic. Report of a WHO consultation on obesity. WHO Press, Geneva
5. Istituto Superiore di Sanità, Stato di attuazione della Legge N. 40/2004, in materia di Procreazione Medicalmente Assistita. 30 aprile 2008, http://www.iss.it/binary/rpma/cont/Ministero%20Salute%20Anno%202007.1214558895.pdf. letto 10 febbraio 2013
6. Pusch H (1996) Environmental factors on male fertility. Fortschr Med 114(14):172–174
7. Sharpe RM (2000) Environment, lifestyle and male infertility. Baillieres Best Pract Res Clin Endocrinol Metab 14(3):489–503
8. Kumar S, Kumari A, Murarka S (2009) Lifestyle factors in deteriorating male reproductive health. Indian J Exp Biol 47(8):615–624
9. Hammoud A, Gibson M, Hunt SC et al (2009) Effect of Roux-en-Y gastric bypass surgery on the sex steroids and quality of life in obese men. J Clin Endocrinol Metab 94(4):1329–1332
10. Schneider G, Kirschner MA, Berkowitz R, Ertel NH (1979) Increased estrogen production in obese men. J Clin Endocrinol Metab 48(4):633–638
11. Akingbemi BT (2005) Estrogen regulation of testicular function. Reprod Biol Endocrinol 3:51
12. Eisenberg ML, Kim S, Chen Z, Sundaram R, Schisterman EF, Buck Louis GM (2014) The relationship between male BMI and waist circumference on semen quality: data from the LIFE study. Hum Reprod 29(2):193–200
13. Jensen TK, Heitmann BL, Jensen MB, Halldorsson TI, Andersson AM, Skakkebæk NE, Joensen UN, Lauritsen MP, Christiansen P, Dalgård C, Lassen TH, Jørgensen N (2013) High dietary intake of saturated fat is associated with reduced semen quality among 701 young Danish men from the general population. Am J Clin Nutr 97(2):411–418
14. Attaman JA, Toth TL, Furtado J, Campos H, Hauser R, Chavarro JE (2012) Dietary fat and semen quality among men attending a fertility clinic. Hum Reprod 27(5):1466–1474
15. Fariello RM, Pariz JR, Spaine DM, Cedenho AP, Bertolla RP, Fraietta R (2012) Association between obesity and alteration of sperm DNA integrity and mitochondrial activity. BJU Int 110(6):863–867
16. Rybar R, Kopecka V, Prinosilova P, Markova P, Rubes J (2011) Male obesity and age in relationship to semen parameters and sperm chromatin integrity. Andrologia 43(4):286–291
17. Martini AC, Tissera A, Estofán D, Molina RI, Mangeaud A, de Cuneo MF, Ruiz RD (2010) Overweight and seminal quality: a study of 794 patients. Fertil Steril 94(5):1739–1743
18. Safarinejad MR (2011) Effect of omega-3 polyunsaturated fatty acid supplementation on semen profile and enzymatic anti-oxidant capacity of seminal plasma in infertile men with idiopathic oligoasthenoteratospermia: a double-blind, placebo-controlled, randomised study. Andrologia 43(1):38–47
19. Chavarro JE, Toth TL, Wright DL, Meeker JD, Hauser R (2010) Body mass index in relation to semen quality, sperm DNA integrity, and serum reproductive hormone levels among men attending an infertility clinic. Fertil Steril 93(7):2222–2231
20. Hofny ER, Ali ME, Abdel-Hafez HZ, Kamal E-D, Mohamed EE, Abd El-Azeem HG, Mostafa T (2010) Semen parameters and hormonal profile in obese fertile and infertile males. Fertil Steril 94(2):581–584
21. Pauli EM, Legro RS, Demers LM, Kunselman AR, Dodson WC, Lee PA (2008) Diminished paternity and gonadal function with increasing obesity in men. Fertil Steril 90(2):346–351
22. Agbaje IM, Rogers DA, McVicar CM, McClure N, Atkinson AB, Mallidis C, Lewis SE (2007) Insulin dependant diabetes mellitus: implications for male reproductive function. Hum Reprod 22(7):1871–1877

23. Fejes I, Koloszár S, Szöllosi J, Závaczki Z, Pál A (2005) Is semen quality affected by male body fat distribution? Andrologia 37(5):155–159
24. Kort HI, Massey JB, Elsner CW et al (2006) Impact of body mass index values on sperm quantity and quality. J Androl 27(3):450–452
25. Jensen TK, Andersson AM, Jørgensen N et al (2004) Body mass index in relation to semen quality and reproductive hormones among 1,558 Danish men. Fertil Steril 82(4):863–870
26. Anderson K, Nisenblat V, Norman R (2010) Lifestyle factors in people seeking infertility treatment – a review. Aust N Z J Obstet Gynaecol 50(1):8–20
27. Lau DC, Douketis JD, Morrison KM, Hramiak IM, Sharma AM, Ur E (2007) 2006 Canadian clinical practice guidelines on the management and prevention of obesity in adults and children. CMAJ 176(8):S1–S13
28. Schlegel PN (2012) Aromatase inhibitors for male infertility. Fertil Steril 98(6):1359–1362
29. Comninos AN, Jayasena CN, Dhillo WS (2014) The relationship between gut and adipose hormones, and reproduction. Hum Reprod Update 20(2):153–174
30. Feeley RJ, Traish AM (2009) Obesity and erectile dysfunction: is androgen deficiency the common link? Sci World J 9:676–684
31. Noblanc A, Kocer A, Chabory E, Vernet P, Saez F, Cadet R, Conrad M, Drevet JR (2011) Glutathione peroxidases at work on epididymal spermatozoa: an example of the dual effect of reactive oxygen species on mammalian male fertilizing ability. J Androl 32(6):641–650
32. Carrell DT (2010) Biology of spermatogenesis and male infertility. Syst Biol Reprod Med 56(3):205–206
33. Balabanič D, Rupnik M, Klemenčič AK (2011) Negative impact of endocrine-disrupting compounds on human reproductive health. Reprod Fertil Dev 23(3):403–416
34. Barazani Y, Katz BF, Nagler HM, Stember DS (2014) Lifestyle, environment, and male reproductive health. Urol Clin North Am 41(1):55–66
35. Keller KB, Lemberg L (2003) Obesity and the metabolic syndrome. Am J Crit Care 12(2):167–170
36. Van Buren DJ, Sinton MM (2009) Psychological aspects of weight loss and weight maintenance. J Am Diet Assoc 109(12):1994–1996
37. Zini A, San Gabriel M, Baazeem A (2009) Antioxidants and sperm DNA damage: a clinical perspective. J Assist Reprod Genet 26(8):427–432
38. Hammoud AO, Meikle AW, Reis LO, Gibson M, Peterson CM, Carrell DT (2012) Obesity and male infertility: a practical approach. Semin Reprod Med 30(6):486–495
39. Moein MR, Tabibnejad N, Ghasemzadeh J (2012) Beneficial effect of tamoxifen on sperm recovery in infertile men with nonobstructive azoospermia. Andrologia 44(Suppl 1):194–198

Unexplained Couple Infertility (Male Role)

11

Giorgio Cavallini

11.1 Definition

Unexplained male infertility (UMI) is defined as infertility whereby semen analysis is normal [1, 2]. Genetic defects are regarded as causes of UMI. Genetically compromised spermatozoa used in assisted reproductive technology (ART) have been associated with a wide range of abnormal embryo development [3]. A proper diagnosis of UMI is mandatory.

11.2 Epidemiology

Failure to determine the cause of infertility occurs in 15 % of infertile couples, which therefore are possibly indicated as UMI [4].

11.3 Etiology

Genetic abnormalities may be associated with UMI [1–3, 5–8] and can be categorized as follows: (1) chromosomal defects in the somatic cells; (2) gene mutations and polymorphisms in the somatic cells; (3) sperm chromosomal abnormalities; and (4) epigenetic disorders.

G. Cavallini
Andrological Section, Gynepro-Medical Team,
via Tranquillo Cremona 8, Bologna 40137, Italy
e-mail: giorgiocavallini@libero.it

11.3.1 Chromosomal Defects

Patients with chromosomal translocation may have different types of alteration of spermatogenesis: from normal spermatogenesis to inability to produce spermatogonia [9]. Chromosomal translocations occur when nonhomologous chromosomes exchange segments. Translocations can be balanced (in an even exchange of material with no genetic information extra or missing, and ideally full functionality) or unbalanced (where the exchange of chromosome material is unequal, resulting in extra or missing genes). Robertsonian translocations (RT) are among the most common balanced structural rearrangements in humans, and comprise complete chromatin fusion of the long arm of two acrocentric chromosomes. RT gives rise to one large metacentric chromosome and one extremely small chromosome that may be lost from the organism with little effect because it contains so few genes. The resulting karyotype in humans leaves only 45 chromosomes, as two chromosomes have fused together. RTs are relatively frequent, and affect fertility in 1 of every 1,000 men [10]. Carriers of RT may exhibit normal phenotype but be otherwise infertile because of more or less severe sperm abnormalities [11]. RT, however, may account for only few cases of unexplained infertility [12].

11.3.2 Gene Mutations

UMI includes mutations of cation channel of sperm (CatSper) and sperm mitochondrial genes. The diagnosis of gene mutations can be made only by molecular genetic testing.

11.3.2.1 CatSper Gene

Voltage-gated calcium channels (CatSper 1–4) and H^+ are four pumps located in the principal part of the sperm flagellum. The action of CatSper in human spermatozoa can induce elevation of both intracellular pH and Ca^{2+} required for sperm activation in the female reproductive tract (hyperactivation) [13, 14] which is positively correlated with the extent of zona pellucida binding, acrosome reaction, zona-free oocyte penetration, and fertilization capacity in vitro [15]. An abnormally low proportion of sperm exhibiting hyperactivation has been found in UMI associated with CatSper1 gene mutations. CatSper-related male infertility is inherited in an autosomal recessive manner [16].

11.3.2.2 Sperm Mitochondrial Deoxyribonucleic Acid Mutations

Sperm mitochondria are located around the mid-segment in a helical arrangement containing mitochondrial deoxyribonucleic acid (mtDNA). mtDNA encodes 37 genes that regulate the Krebs cycle (oxidative phosphorylation). mtDNA is not protected by histones and physically associates with the inner mitochondrial membrane, where highly mutagenic oxygen radicals are generated by the respiratory chain [17, 18]. Thus mtDNA is more prone than nuclear DNA to mutations.

Mitochondrial DNA polymerase gamma (POLG) is a key reparative enzyme of mDNA strands that encode for the POLG gene. The POLG gene is associated with UMI [19, 20].

11.3.3 Sperm Chromosomal Abnormalities

A threefold increase in the frequency of sperm aneuploidy is found in infertile men (approximately 3 %) in comparison with their fertile counterparts [21]. Sperm aneuploidy has been associated with severe sperm defects, UMI, recurrent miscarriage, failure of in vitro fertilization, and increased risk of chromosome abnormalities in newborns [21, 22].

11.3.4 Epigenetic Disorders

Epigenetics defines all types of molecular information (independent of DNA) transmitted from the spermatozoa to the embryo. The epigenetic regulatory mechanisms include, in theory: (1) centrosome; (2) DNA methylation; (3) histone modifications; (4) chromatin remodeling; and (5) role of RNA transcripts.

Histone covalent modifications are associated with several nuclear functions including transcriptional control, chromatin packaging, and DNA methylation. If abnormally modified, histones might impede normal embryogenesis [23, 24]. It is thought that assessments of DNA condensation/decondensation or fluorescent in situ hybridization of sperm chromosomes might be useful tools for these patients, although the poor reproducibility of tests raises doubts about their clinical usefulness [23, 24].

11.3.5 Germ Cell Splicing Factor

Alternative splicing of precursor messenger RNA (pre-mRNA) is common in mammalian cells and enables the production of multiple gene products from a single gene, thus increasing transcriptome and proteome diversity. Disturbance of splicing regulation is associated with many human diseases; however, key splicing factors that control tissue-specific alternative splicing remain largely undefined. In an unbiased genetic screen for essential male fertility genes in the mouse, the author's group identified the RNA-binding protein RBM5 (RNA binding motif 5) as an essential regulator of haploid male germ cell pre-mRNA splicing and fertility. This gene encodes several apoptosis-related proteins including *Caspase 2* [25], *FAS* receptor, and *c-FLIP* [26]. It has been suggested that RBM5 male germ cell splicing factor is one of the contributory factors in UMI [27].

11.3.6 Chromosome Heteromorphism

Certain regions in the genome are subject to heteromorphisms because of their repetitive DNA content. Chromosome localizations of these regions may be identified by several methods, each of which reveals typical staining patterns implying constitutional differences in heterochromatin [28]. The term heteromorphism is used synonymously with the polymorphism or normal variant. Common cytogenetic polymorphisms detected by G-banding are considered as heteromorphisms

Table 11.1 Genetic tests in unexplained male infertility [30, 31]

Test	Objective	Specimen tested
Cytogenetic test	Assess number and appearance of chromosomes	Blood
Gene sequencing	Determine gene sequencing for mutations	Blood
Fluorescence in situ hybridization	Assess spermatozoa aploidy	Sperm
Microarray technology	Analyze copy number variations, gene expression levels, single-nucleotide polymorphisms, and mRNA transcripts pool expressed by sperm	Sperm, blood
Next-generation sequencing technologies	Detect DNA mutilation problems	Blood
Giemsa-trypsin banding (G-banding)	Detect chromosome polymorphism	Blood

and include heterochromatin regions of chromosomes 1, 9, 16, and Y, and also prominent acrocentric short arms, satellites, and stalks [29]. There seems to be an increased incidence, especially in UMI men, but the mechanism underlying this association needs to be elucidated [30].

11.4 Diagnosis

A series of tests can be used to identify genetic and epigenetic defects in UMI (Table 11.1) [30, 31]. Unfortunately, these tests are not routinely available. Despite being limited by the widespread use of ART, a cost-effective genetic evaluation should be considered as an integral part of the workup in UMI. POLG gene mutations can be detected using sequence analysis, and testing is clinically available (www.transgenomic.com).

11.5 Therapy

At present the only available therapy is ART. Of note, the prognosis for pregnancy by POLG gene alterations is good in cases treated with ART, as mtDNA is not transmitted to the offspring [11]. About one-half of the couples submitted to ART are affected by UMI. In the author's opinion frustration induced by infertility, notwithstanding laboratory examinations within the reference values, might play a critical role on the behavior of these couples.

References

1. Hamada A, Esteves SC, Nizza M, Agarwal A (2012) Unexplained male infertility: diagnosis and management. Int Braz J Urol 38:576–594

2. Sigman M, Lipshultz L, Howard S (2009) Office evaluation of the subfertile male. In: Lipshultz LI, Howards SS, Niederberger CS (eds) Infertility in the male, 4th edn. Cambridge University Press, Cambridge, pp 153–176
3. Aitken RJ, Koopman P, Lewis SE (2004) Seeds of concern. Nature 432:48–52
4. Esteves SC, Zini A, Aziz N, Alvarez JG, Sabanegh ES Jr, Agarwal A (2012) Critical appraisal of world health organization's new reference values for human semen characteristics and effect on diagnosis and treatment of subfertile men. Urology 79:16–22
5. Hamada A, Esteves SC, Agarwal A (2012) Genetics and male infertility. In: Dubey AK (ed) Infertility, diagnosis, management and IVF, 1st edn. Jaypee Medical Publishers Inc., New Delhi, pp 113–157
6. Bailey JA, Gu Z, Clark RA, Reinert K, Samonte RV, Schwartz S (2002) Recent segmental duplications in the human genome. Science 297:1003–1007
7. Hargreave TB (2000) Genetic basis of male fertility. Br Med Bull 56:650–671
8. Matzuk MM, Lamb DJ (2002) Genetic dissection of mammalian fertility pathways. Nat Cell Biol 4:41–49
9. Georgiou I, Syrrou M, Pardalidis N, Karakitsios K, Mantzavinos T, Giotitsas N et al (2006) Genetic and epigenetic risks of intracytoplasmic sperm injection method. Asian J Androl 8:643–673
10. Ferlin A, Raicu F, Gatta V, Zuccarello D, Palka G, Foresta C (2007) Male infertility: role of genetic background. Reprod Biomed Online 14:734–745
11. Dada R, Thilagavathi J, Venkatesh S, Esteves SC, Agarwal A (2011) Genetic testing in male infertility. Open Reprod Sci J 3:42–56
12. Conn CM, Cozzi J, Harper JC, Winston RM, Delhanty JD (1999) Preimplantation genetic diagnosis for couples at high risk of Down syndrome pregnancy owing to parental translocation or mosaicism. J Med Genet 36:45–50
13. Lishko PV, Kirichok Y (2010) The role of Hv1 and CatSper channels in sperm activation. J Physiol 588:4667–4672
14. Carlson AE, Burnett LA, del Camino D, Quill TA, Hille B, Chong JA (2009) Pharmacological targeting of native CatSper channels reveals a required role in maintenance of sperm hyperactivation. PLoS One 4:e6844
15. Esteves SC, Verza S Jr (2011) Relationship of *in vitro* acrosome reaction to sperm function: an update. Open Reprod Sci J 3:72–84
16. Hildebrand MS, Avenarius MR, Fellous M, Zhang Y, Meyer NC, Auer J (2010) Genetic male infertility and mutation of CATSPER ion channels. Eur J Hum Genet 18:1178–1184
17. Venkatesh S, Deecaraman M, Kumar R, Shamsi MB, Dada R (2009) Role of reactive oxygen species in the pathogenesis of mitochondrial DNA (mtDNA) mutations in male infertility. Indian J Med Res 129:127–137
18. Richter C, Suter M, Walter PB (1998) Mitochondrial free radical damage and DNA repair. Biofactors 7:207–208
19. Rovio AT, Marchington DR, Donat S, Schuppe HC, Abel J, Fritsche E (2001) Mutations at the mitochondrial DNA polymerase (POLG) locus associated with male infertility. Nat Genet 29:261–262
20. Jensen M, Leffers H, Petersen JH, Nyboe Andersen A, Jørgensen N, Carlsen E (2004) Frequent polymorphism of the mitochondrial DNA polymerase gamma gene (POLG) in patients with normal spermiograms and unexplained subfertility. Hum Reprod 19:65–70
21. Moosani N, Pattinson HA, Carter MD, Cox DM, Rademaker AW, Martin RH (1995) Chromosomal analysis of sperm from men with idiopathic infertility using sperm karyotyping and fluorescence *in situ* hybridization. Fertil Steril 64:811–817
22. Tempest HG, Martin RH (2009) Cytogenetic risks in chromosomally normal infertile men. Curr Opin Obstet Gynecol 21:223–227
23. Carrell DT, Emery BR, Hammoud S (2007) Altered protamine expression and diminished spermatogenesis: what is the link? Hum Reprod Update 13:313–327
24. Nanassy L, Carrell DT (2008) Paternal effects on early embryogenesis. J Exp Clin Assist Reprod 5:2

25. Fushimi K, Ray P, Kar A, Wang L, Sutherland LC et al (2008) Up-regulation of the proapoptotic caspase 2 splicing isoform by a candidate tumor suppressor, RBM5. Proc Natl Acad Sci U S A 105:15708–15713. doi:10.1073/pnas.0805569105
26. Bonnal S, Martinez C, Forch P, Bachi A, Wilm M et al (2008) RBM5/Luca-15/H37 regulates Fas alternative splice site pairing after exon definition. Mol Cell 32:81–95
27. O'Bryan MK, Clark BJ, McLaughlin EA, D'Sylva RJ, O'Donnell L et al (2013) RBM5 is a male germ cell splicing factor and is required for spermatid differentiation and male fertility. PLoS Genet 9(7):e1003628
28. Babu A, Agarwal AK, Verma S (1998) A new approach in recognition of heterochromatic regions of human chromosomes by means of restriction endonucleases. Am J Hum Genet 42:60–65
29. Brothman AR, Schneider NR, Saikevych I, Cooley LD, Butler MG, Patil S, Mascarello JT, Rao KW, Dewald GW, Park JP, Persons DL, Wolff DJ, Vance GH, Cytogenetics Resource Committee, College of American Pathologists/American College of Medical Genetics (2006) Cytogenetic heteromorphisms: survey results and reporting practices of giemsa-band regions that we have pondered for years. Arch Pathol Lab Med 130:947–949
30. Sahin FI, Yilmaz Z, Yuregir OO, Bulakbasi T, Ozer O, Zeyneloglu HB (2008) Chromosome heteromorphisms: an impact on infertility. J Assist Reprod Genet 25:191–195
31. Esteves SC (2013) A clinical appraisal of the genetic basis in unexplained male infertility. J Hum Reprod Sci 6:176–182

Inflammatory Infertility

12

Giorgio Cavallini and Gianni Paulis

12.1 Definition

Inflammatory infertility occurs when male infertility is provoked by inflammation of the urogenital tract and might constitute a curable cause of infertility [1]. About 10–15 % of infertile men have genital tract inflammation. After exclusion of urethritis and/or bladder infection, a sperm leukocyte concentration of $>10^6$/mL indicates inflammation [2]. It was recently advocated that a high leukocyte count in prostate-specific materials, even in the absence of clear leukocytospermia, may be associated with male infertility/dyspermia [3]. A concentration of $>10^3$ colony-forming units is significant for bacteriospermia [2].

Clinical studies raise doubts about whether inflammation of epididymis and didymis negatively affect male fertility when seminal duct obstruction is absent [4], leading to the suspicion that inflammation of the testicles exerts a poor influence on fertility. In fact, inflammation is one of the most important components of immune protection. On coming into contact with pathogen antigens, cells of the inflammatory response release signaling molecules (proinflammatory cytokines), which amplify the response by recruiting other macrophages and granulocytes to the infection site. To prevent inflammatory damage, another set of signaling molecules have the function of turning the signal off [5]. However, the disruption of immune response at the testicular level strongly affects spermatogenesis, indicating a protective role of the immune system in regard of fertility potential [6, 7].

G. Cavallini (✉)
Andrological Section, Gynepro-Medical Team,
via Tranquillo Cremona 8, Bologna 40137, Italy
e-mail: giorgiocavallini@libero.it

G. Paulis
Department of Urology, Andrology Center, Regina Apostolorum Hospital, Albano L., Rome, Italy
e-mail: paulisg@libero.it

Further testicular macrophages play an important role in the balance between defense against invading microorganisms and "testicular immune privilege," which serves to protect the neoantigens of the meiotic and haploid germ cells that appear during puberty after the establishment of self-tolerance. Although testicular macrophages exhibit many typical macrophage characteristics such as effective antigen presentation, phagocytic functions, and expression of Fc receptors and major histocompatibility complex class II receptor [8], they are more reminiscent of a type-2 macrophage displaying diminished proinflammatory responses and reduced capacity to induce T-cell activation [9].

Thus the majority of the so-called inflammatory infertilities are of prostatic origin, with epididymitis of marginal interest.

12.2 Epididymitis

Acute epididymitis is divided into two classes [10, 11].

1. Sexually transmitted epididymitis (usually linked to urethritis), caused most often by *Neisseria gonorrhoeae* or *Chlamydia trachomatis*, occurs among sexually active adults younger than 35 years
2. Nonsexually transmitted epididymitis is often associated with urinary tract infections, and occurs more often in adults older than 35 or who have recently undergone urinary instrumentation procedures

A slight impairment of sperm forward motility might occur, which is completely recovered after appropriate antibiotic therapy [12]. Obstructive azoospermia after bilateral epididymitis can occur, although its prevalence is unknown.

12.3 Prostatitis

12.3.1 Definition and Categorization

Prostatitis is a prostatic inflammation. About half of all men suffer from prostatitis symptoms during their life span [13, 14]. Prostatitis is classified according to five categories: acute prostatitis (category I), chronic bacterial prostatitis (category II), abacterial inflammatory prostatitis (category IIIa), abacterial noninflammatory prostatitis (category IIIb), and asymptomatic prostatitis (category IV) [15].

Chronic prostatitis increases the risk for benign prostatic hyperplasia and prostate cancer [16, 17], and may affect male reproductive health [18].

12.3.2 Etiology of Prostatitis

Escherichia coli, *Klebsiella* sp., *Proteus mirabilis*, *Enterococcus faecalis*, *Pseudomonas aeruginosa*, *C. trachomatis*, and *Ureaplasma urealiticum* are the most common bacteria involved in bacterial prostatitis infections. The route of infection is urinary ascending or lymphatic transrectal [19].

12.3.3 Pathogenesis of Dyspermia Associated with Prostatitis

Most of the literature agrees that the existence of bacteria in the prostate is linked with asthenospermia and decreased male reproductive health [20]. Chronic prostatitis seems to affect sperm count mainly if associated with irritable bowel syndrome, because of dilation of the periprostatic venous plexus and increased temperature [21]. An increase in reactive oxygen species (ROS) from leukocytes [22] has been indicated as a further physiopathologic mechanism of dyspermia associated with prostatitis.

12.3.4 Diagnosis

Although several symptomatic indices for prostatitis have been developed, only the National Institutes of Health (NIH) Chronic Prostatitis Collaborative Research Network has produced a valid instrument for evaluation of symptoms of prostatitis: the NIH Chronic Prostatitis Symptom Index (NIH-CPSI). This index has nine items divided into three domains (pain, urinary symptoms, and quality of life), and is used as a tool for the diagnosis and follow-up of chronic prostatitis and chronic pelvic pain syndrome. Initially it was presented in English [23] (Table 12.1) and later also in Italian [24].

The prostate is tender, with various degrees of pain at objective examination. Urine culture and expressed prostatic secretion (EPS) represent the most important investigations for the diagnosis and categorization of prostatitis. EPS has been fully described by Mears and Stamey (Table 12.2) [25].

If prostatic biopsy is contraindicated [26], transrectal echography might be of some help when stones or abscess are suspected [27]. The efficacy of semen culture in the diagnosis and evaluation of chronic prostatitis remains unclear, and ejaculate culture is not recommended as a first line of diagnostic evaluation in these patients [28]. Increased seminal plasma elastase [1], interleukins (especially interleukin-6) [29], and ROS [1], in addition to decreased zinc, citric acid, fructose, phosphatase, and α-glutamyltransferase [30], are regarded as biochemical signs of chronic prostatitis.

Table 12.1 National Institutes of Health Chronic Prostatitis Symptom Index (NIH-CPSI) [23]
Part a: National institutes of Health: classification system for prostatitis

Type		Classification	Definition
I		Acute bacterial prostatitis	Evidence of acute bacterial infection
II		Chronic bacterial prostatits	Evidence of recurrent bacterial infection
III	A	Chronic abacterial inflammatory prostatitis	White blood cells in semen, expressed prostatic secretions or VB3
	B	Chronic abacterial non-inflammatory prostatitis	No white blood cells in semen, expressed prostatic secretions or VB3
IV		Asymptomatic inflammatory prostatits	No symptoms, incidental diagnosis during prostate biopsy or presence of white blood cells in prostatic secretions during evaluation for others disorders.

Part b) NIH Chronic Prostatitis Symptom Index (NIH-CPSI).

Pain or discomfort.
1) In the last week, have you experienced any pain or discomfort in the following areas?

	Yes	No
a) Area between rectum and testicles (perineum)	1	0
b) Testicles	1	0
c) Tip of the penis (not related to urination)	1	0
d) Below your waist, in your pubic or bladder area	1	0

2) In the last week, have you experienced:

	Yes	No
a) Pain or burning during urination	1	0
b) Pain or discomfort during or after sexual climax (ejaculation)	1	0

3) How often have you had pain or discomfort in any of these areas over the last week?

0	Never
1	Rarely
2	Sometimes
3	Often
4	Usually
5	Always

4) Which number best describes your average pain or discomfort on the days that you had it, over the last week? 0 = no pain; 10 = pain as bad you can imagine.

0	1	2	3	4	5	6	7	8	9	10

Urination
5) How often have you had a sensation of not emptying your bladder completely after you finished urinating over the last week?

0	Not at all
1	Less than 1 time in 5
2	Less than half time
3	About half time

Table 12.1 (continued)

4	More than half time
5	Almost always

6) How often have you had to urinate again less than two hours after after you finished urinating over the last week?

0	Not at all
1	Less than 1 time in 5
2	Less than half time
3	About half time
4	More than half time
5	Almost always

Impact of symptoms

7) How much have your symptoms kept you from doing the kinds of things you would usually do, over the last week?

0	None
1	Only a little
2	Some
3	A lot

8) How much did you think about your symptoms, over the last week?

0	None
1	Only a little
2	Some
3	A lot

Quality of life.

9) If you were to spend the rest of your life with your symptoms just the way they have been during the last week, how would you feel about that?

0	Delighted
1	Pleased
2	Mostly satisfied
3	Mixed (about equally satisfied and dissatisfied)
4	Mostly dissatisfied
5	Unhappy
6	Terrible

Scoring the NIH-Chronic Prostatitis Symptom Index Domains.
Pain: Total of items 1, 2, 3 and 4 =..
Urinary symptoms: Total of items 5 and 6 = ...
Quality of life impact: Total of items 7, 8 and 9................................

Table 12.2 Mears and Stamey localization technique [25]

The test begins when the patient needs to void: drink 500 mL water, 30–60 min before the test
Four sterile containers are needed, named VB1, VB2, EPS, and VB3
Retract completely the foreskin
Cleanse the glans with sterile physiologic solution and dry the glans with sterile gauze
Urinate 10–20 mL in VB1
Urinate 200 mL in the toilet and without interrupting the stream urinate in VB2
The physician massages the prostate until several drops of prostatic secretion are obtained (EPS)
If no EPS could be collected during massage, a drop may be present at the orifice of urethra, and this drop should be taken with a 10-μL calibrated loop and cultured
Immediately after massage the patients urinates 10–15 mL in VB3

12.3.5 Therapy

A full review of the therapy of prostatitis is presented on the Web site of the European Urological Association (EUA): http://www.uroweb.org/guidelines/online-guidelines/?no_cache=1 It should be noted that trimethoprim-sulfamethoxazole is contraindicated for the treatment of inflammatory infertility linked to prostatitis because this drug is toxic for male gametes (see the Chap. 15). The therapy of prostatitis is mainly aimed at resolving the symptoms (see the following paragraph), and from a reproductive point of view the goals are reduction/eradication of microorganisms in prostatic secretions and semen, normalization of sperm inflammatory parameters, and improvement of sperm count [1, 14, 31]. At present only antibiotic therapy is achieving these goals [1].

12.3.6 Prognosis of Prostatitis in Terms of Human Fertility

EUA guidelines indicate that antibiotic treatment often eradicates microorganisms but cannot reverse anatomic dysfunctions, and might improve sperm quality, which does not necessarily enhance the probability of conception [4].

These data are not surprising, because the relationship between male fecundity and sperm count is hyperbolic and achieves a plateau at about 30×10^6 spermatozoa/mL, 50 % class A motility, and 14 % typical forms (strict criteria) [32–34]. Thus the more severe the dyspermia the more crucial is its therapy to improve couple fertility, and chronic prostatitis is seldom associated with severe dyspermia [4, 20, 21]. Furthermore, male fecundity is linked more to the quality of spermatogenesis than to sperm count [35, 36], and spermatogenesis is obviously not or poorly affected in the course of prostatitis. Despite these limitations to therapy, it is generally recognized that appropriate therapy for prostatitis should be performed to ensure, at the very least, symptom relief.

12.4 Mumps Orchitis

Mumps orchitis is rare; however, because of its detrimental sequelae on sperm count it merits discussion here. Orchitis is a common complication of mumps in postpubertal men affecting about 20–30 % of cases (10–30 % of which are bilateral), often results in testicular atrophy, and occurs 1–2 weeks after parotitis [37].

The causes of testicular atrophy are not fully known. In the course of inflammation the tunica albuginea forms a barrier against edema, and the subsequent rise in intratesticular pressure leads to pressure-induced testicular atrophy [38]. Adamopoulos et al. found elevated luteinizing hormone (LH) levels and an exaggerated pituitary response to LH-releasing hormone (LHRH) stimulation in the acute phase of mumps orchitis. Basal testosterone concentrations returned to normal after several months, whereas mean basal follicle-stimulating hormone (FSH) and LH concentrations remained significantly increased at 10 and 12 months after the acute phase [39].

Mumps orchitis rarely leads to azoospermia, more frequently leading to various degrees of dyspermia [40]. Testicular sperm extraction is indicated in cases of azoospermia (even with high concentrations of FSH and LH), whereas no treatment has been proposed for dyspermia [41].

12.5 Sperm DNA Fragmentation in Inflammatory Infertility: A Less Orthodox Point of View

Sperm DNA fragmentation (SDF) is the separation or breaking of DNA strands into pieces. Any form of DNA damage may result in male infertility. Sperm DNA integrity is essential for the complete transmission of genetic information, and is necessary for the normal fertilization and embryo growth in both natural and assisted conception [42, 43], but also for normal fetal development [44]. It has been reported that when 30 % or more of sperm DNA is damaged, natural pregnancy is not possible [45, 46]. Approximately 15 % of patients with male factor infertility have a normal semen analysis [47].

Increased sperm DNA fragmentation is frequently observed in males with normal semen characteristics. In fact, sperm DNA damage is found in 8 % of men with normal seminal parameters [48, 49]. Moreover, a significant proportion of males (8.4–23 %) diagnosed as unexplained infertile according to conventional semen analysis have high levels of sperm DNA fragmentation [50–53]. DNA integrity can be considered an effective monitor of normal male fertility potential [54].

High levels of sperm DNA fragmentation have been correlated with low fertility potential, failure to obtain blastocysts, hindrance in embryonic development, increased risk of recurrent miscarriages, reduced chances of successful implantation, and abnormal outcomes in the offspring [55–57].

Several etiologic factors have been associated with sperm DNA fragmentation: environmental conditions and cigarette smoking [58, 59], chemotherapy [60–62], irradiation [63, 64], cancer [65], varicocele [66, 67], leukocytospermia [68, 69], advanced paternal age [70–72], high fever [73], and chronic prostatitis [74–78]. Sharma et al. found the highest levels of ROS in semen of infertile men with prostatitis [79]. High levels of ROS mediate the DNA fragmentation commonly observed in spermatozoa of infertile men [80, 81]. Therefore, inflammations of the male genitourinary tract can adversely affect male fertility by causing sperm DNA damage.

Chronic prostatitis affects about 10–15 % of the male population [82]. In other studies the prevalence of prostatitis symptoms ranged from 2 to 9.7 % [83–85]. Prostatitis is the most frequent urologic diagnosis in males younger than 50 years [86]. It has been estimated that approximately 50 % of men will suffer from prostatitis during their lifetime [87]. A study of National Center for Health Statistics showed that about 25 % of outpatients evaluated for genitourinary problems suffered from prostatitis [88]. Males with a previous diagnosis of prostatitis had a 20–50 % risk for recurrent episodes [89]. A history of male genital inflammations, including prostatitis, epididymitis, and orchitis, occurs in 5–12 % of infertile men [90].

A study by El-Bayoumi et al. has revealed that prostatitis was the cause of infertility in 27.5 % of a sample of 375 infertile male patients [91]. A more recent study has shown chronic prostatitis as a cause of infertility in 39.1 % of 534 patients with male infertility [92].

Hu et al., in their recent (2013) study, have shown that chronic prostatitis significantly reduces sperm quality and male fertility, also highlighting a significant increase in sperm DNA fragmentation [76].

Considering that sperm DNA fragmentation is a frequent condition (due to various causes) and that chronic prostatitis is also very common and causes infertility in a high percentage of cases, one can deduce that sperm DNA damage is a frequent precondition for male infertility.

As sperm DNA fragmentation cannot be detected by routine molecular and cytogenetic methods, several assays have been developed to evaluate sperm chromatin/DNA integrity.

Some of these tests measure DNA damage directly, such as TUNEL (terminal deoxynucleotidyl transferase-mediated deoxyuridine triphosphate nick-end labeling assay) and COMET (single-cell gel electrophoresis) [93, 94]. Other tests (indirect) include SCSA (sperm chromatin structure assay) and the SCD test (sperm chromatin dispersion) [95, 96]. The SCD test and TUNEL assay are both effective in detecting sperm DNA damage; however, using bright-field microscopy, the SCD test appears to be more sensitive than TUNEL [97]. Sperm DNA fragmentation has now become a new biomarker for male infertility diagnosis [98].

There are several notable facts regarding the interpretation and evaluation of the results of these different methods, as follows.

SCSA: The pregnancy rates are significantly higher with DNA fragmentation index (DFI) below the thresholds of 30–40 % [99]. Other investigators have found that a DFI cutoff level of 30.27 % was able to discriminate infertile and fertile men [100];

TUNEL: A threshold value of 20 % sperm DNA fragmentation (SDF) has been suggested to distinguish between fertile men and infertile patients [54]. A more recent study has shown a cutoff value of 19.2 % that can differentiate infertile men with DNA damage from healthy men [101];
COMET (alkaline test): The risk of failure to achieve a pregnancy increases when SDF exceeds a prognostic threshold value of 52 % [102];
COMET (neutral test): When SDF exceeds a prognostic threshold value of 77.5 %, there is a high risk of pregnancy failure [103];
SCD test: Men with SDF greater than a diagnostic threshold of 22.75 have a high risk of infertility [103].

According to current knowledge, intake of antioxidants may be beneficial in reducing sperm DNA damage, particularly in men with high levels of DNA fragmentation [104]. It is also important to identify behaviors that may reduce sperm DNA damage, such as removing testicular gonadotoxins and/or hyperthermia, treatment of genital tract infections and chronic prostatitis, correction of varicocele, smoking cessation, and reducing radiation exposure [80, 104–109].

References

1. Weidner W, Krause W, Ludwig M (1999) Relevance of male accessory gland infection for subsequent fertility with special focus on prostatitis. Hum Reprod Update 5:421–432
2. World Health Organization (2010) WHO manual for the examination and processing of human semen, 5th edn. Cambridge University Press, Cambridge
3. Punab M, Kullisaar T, Mändar R (2013) Male infertility workup needs additional testing of expressed prostatic secretion and/or post-massage urine. PLoS One 8(12):e82776
4. Jungwirth A, Giwercman A, Tournaye H, Diemer T, Kopa Z, Dohle G, Krausz C, European Association of Urology Working Group on Male Infertility (2012) European Association of Urology guidelines on Male Infertility: the 2012 update. Eur Urol 62:324–332
5. Max EE, Sell S (2001) Immunology, immunopathology, and immunity. ASM Press, Washington, DC
6. Belloni V, Sorci G, Paccagnini E, Guerreiro R, Bellenger J, Faivre B (2014) Disrupting immune regulation incurs transient costs in male reproductive function. PLoS One 9(1):e84606. doi:10.1371/journal.pone.0084606
7. Mayerhofer A (2013) Human testicular peritubular cells: more than meets the eye. Reproduction 145:107–116
8. Hedger MP (2002) Macrophages and the immune responsiveness of the testis. J Reprod Immunol 57:19–34
9. Bhushan S, Hossain H, Lu Y, Geisler A, Tchatalbachev S, Mikulski Z, Schuler G, Klug J, Pilatz A, Wagenlehner F, Chakraborty T, Meinhardt A (2011) Uropathogenic E. coli induce different immune response in testicular and peritoneal macrophages: implications for testicular immune privilege. PLoS One 6(12):e28452
10. Berger RE, Alexander ER, Harnisch JP, Paulsen CA, Monda GD, Ansell J, Holmes KK (1979) Etiology, manifestations and therapy of acute epididymitis: prospective study of 50 cases. J Urol 121:750–754
11. Trojian TH, Lishnak TS, Heiman D (2009) Epididymitis and orchitis: an overview. Am Fam Physician 79:583–587
12. Centers for Disease Control and Prevention. Sexually transmitted diseases. Treatment guidelines 2006. Epididymitis. http://www.cdc.gov/std/treatment/2006/epididymitis
13. Domingue GJ Sr, Hellstrom WJ (1998) Prostatitis. Clin Microbiol Rev 11:604–613
14. Schaeffer AJ (2006) Clinical practice. Chronic prostatitis and the chronic pelvic pain syndrome. N Engl J Med 355:1690–1698
15. Nickel JC (2003) Prostatitis: diagnosis and classification. Curr Urol Rep 4:259–260
16. Cheng I, Witte JS, Jacobsen SJ, Haque R, Quinn VP, Quesenberry CP, Caan BJ, Van Den Eeden SK (2010) Prostatitis, sexually transmitted diseases, and prostate cancer: the California Men's Health Study. PLoS One 5:e8736
17. Krieger JN, Riley DE, Cheah PY, Liong ML, Yuen KH (2003) Epidemiology of prostatitis: new evidence for a world-wide problem. World J Urol 21:70–74
18. Lobel B, Rodriguez A (2003) Chronic prostatitis: what we know, what we do not know, and what we should do! World J Urol 21:57–63
19. Choi YS, Kim KS, Choi SW, Kim S, Bae WJ, Cho HJ, Hong SH, Kim SW, Hwang TK, Lee JY (2013) Microbiological etiology of bacterial prostatitis in general hospital and primary care clinic in Korea. Prostate Int 1:133–138
20. Hou DS, Long WM, Shen J, Zhao LP, Pang XY, Xu C (2012) Characterisation of the bacterial community in expressed prostatic secretions from patients with chronic prostatitis/chronic pelvic pain syndrome and infertile men: a preliminary investigation. Asian J Androl 14:566–573
21. Vicari E, La Vignera S, Arcoria D, Condorelli R, Vicari LO, Castiglione R, Mangiameli A, Calogero AE (2011) High frequency of chronic bacterial and non-inflammatory prostatitis in infertile patients with prostatitis syndrome plus irritable bowel syndrome. PLoS One 6(4):e18647

22. Walczak-Jedrzejowska R, Wolski JK, Slowikowska-Hilczer J (2013) The role of oxidative stress and antioxidants in male fertility. Cent European J Urol 66:60–67
23. Litwin MS, McNaughton-Collins M, Fowler FJ Jr, Nickel JC, Calhoun EA, Pontari MA, Alexander RB, Farrar JT, O'Leary MP (1999) The National Institutes of Health chronic prostatitis symptom index: development and validation of a new outcome measure. Chronic Prostatitis Collaborative Research Network. J Urol 162:369–375
24. Giubilei G, Mondaini N, Crisci A, Raugei A, Lombardi G, Travaglini F, Del Popolo G, Bartoletti R (2005) The Italian version of the National Institutes of Health Chronic Prostatitis Symptom Index. Eur Urol 47:805–811
25. Mears EM, Stamey TAS (1969) Bacteriologic localization patterns in bacterial prostatitis and ureteritis. Invest Urol 5:492–518
26. Oh MM, Chae JY, Kim JW, Kim JW, Yoon CY, Park MG, du Moon G (2013) Positive culture for extended-spectrum β-lactamase during acute prostatitis after prostate biopsy is a risk factor for progression to chronic prostatitis. Urology 81:1209–1212
27. Shoskes DA, Lee CT, Murphy D, Kefer J, Wood HM (2007) Incidence and significance of prostatic stones in men with chronic prostatitis/chronic pelvic pain syndrome. Urology 70:235–238
28. Lee KS, Choi JD (2012) Chronic prostatitis: approaches for best management. Korean J Urol 53:69–77
29. Dousset B, Hussenet F, Daudin M, Bujan L, Foliguet B, Nabet P (1997) Seminal cytokine concentrations (IL-1beta, IL-2, IL-6, sR IL-2, sR IL-6), semen parameters and blood hormonal status in male infertility. Hum Reprod 12:1476–1479
30. Comhaire F, Verschraegen G, Vermeulen L (1980) Diagnosis of accessory gland infection and its possible role in male infertility. Int J Androl 3:32–45
31. Wagenlehner FM, Diemer T, Naber KG, Weidner W (2008) Chronic bacterial prostatitis (NIH type II): diagnosis, therapy and influence on the fertility status. Andrologia 40:100–104
32. Bonde JP, Ernst E, Jensen TK, Hjollund NH, Kolstad H, Henriksen TB, Scheike T, Giwercman A, Olsen J, Skakkebaek NE (1998) Relation between semen quality and fertility: a population-based study of 430 first-pregnancy planners. Lancet 352:1172–1177
33. Cooper TG, Noonan E, von Eckardstein S, Auger J, Baker HW, Behre HM, Haugen TB, Kruger T, Wang C, Mbizvo MT, Vogelsong KM (2010) World Health Organization reference values for human semen characteristics. Hum Reprod Update 16:231–245
34. Guzick DS, Overstreet JW, Factor-Litvak P, Brazil CK, Nakajima ST, Coutifaris C, Carson SA, Cisneros P, Steinkampf MP, Hill JA, Xu D, Vogel DL, National Cooperative Reproductive Medicine Network (2001) Sperm morphology, motility, and concentration in fertile and infertile men. N Engl J Med 345:1388–1393
35. Cavallini G, Cristina Magli M, Crippa A, Resta S, Vitali G, Pia Ferraretti A, Gianaroli L (2011) The number of spermatozoa collected with testicular sperm extraction is a novel predictor of intracytoplasmic sperm injection outcome in non-obstructive azoospermic patients. Asian J Androl 13:312–316
36. Cavallini G, Magli MC, Crippa A, Ferraretti AP, Gianaroli L (2012) Reduction in sperm aneuploidy levels in severe oligoasthenoteratospermic patients after medical therapy: a preliminary report. Asian J Androl 14:591–598
37. Masarani M, Wazait H, Dinneen M (2006) Mumps orchitis. J R Soc Med 99:573–575
38. Bartak V (1973) Sperm count, morphology, and motility after unilateral mumps orchitis. J Reprod Fertil 32:491–493
39. Adamopoulos DA, Lawrence DM, Vassilopoulos P, Contoyiannis PA, Swyer GI (1978) Pituitary-testicular interrelationships in mumps orchitis and other infections. BMJ 1:1177–1180
40. Casella R, Leibundgut B, Lehmann K, Gasser TC (1997) Mumps orchitis: report of a mini-epidemic. J Urol 158:2158–2161
41. Masuda H, Inamoto T, Azuma H, Katsuoka Y, Tawara F (2011) Successful testicular sperm extraction in an azoospermic man with postpubertal mumps orchitis. Hinyokika Kiyo 57:529–530

42. Agarwal A, Said TM (2003) Role of sperm chromatin abnormalities and DNA damage in male infertility. Hum Reprod Update 9:331–345
43. De Jonge C (2002) The clinical value of sperm nuclear DNA assessment. Hum Fertil 5:51–53
44. Morris ID, Ilott S, Dixon L, Brison DR (2002) The spectrum of DNA damage in human sperm assessed by single cell gel electrophoresis (Comet assay) and its relationship to fertilization and embryo development. Hum Reprod 17:990–998
45. Evenson DP, Larson KL, Jost LK (2002) Sperm chromatin structure assay: its clinical use for detecting sperm DNA fragmentation in male infertility and comparisons with the other techniques. J Androl 23:25–43
46. Evenson DP, Jost LK, Marshall D et al (1999) Utility of sperm chromatin structure assay as a diagnostic and prognostic tool in the human fertility clinic. Hum Reprod 14:1039–1049
47. Agarwal A, Allamaneni SS (2005) Sperm DNA damage assessment: a test whose time has come. Fertil Steril 84:850–853
48. Zini A, Bielecki R, Phang D et al (2001) Correlations between two markers of sperm DNA integrity, DNA denaturation and DNA fragmentation, in fertile and infertile men. Fertil Steril 75:674–677
49. Zini A, Kamal K, Phang D et al (2001) Biologic variability of sperm DNA denaturation in infertile men. Urology 58:258–261
50. Oleszczuk K, Augustinsson L, Bayat N et al (2013) Prevalence of high DNA fragmentation index in male partners of unexplained infertile couples. Andrology 1(3):357–360
51. Qiu Y, Wang L, Zhang L et al (2008) Analysis of sperm chromosomal abnormalities and sperm DNA fragmentation in infertile males. Zhonghua Yi Xue Yi Chuan Xue Za Zhi 25(6):681–685
52. Host E, Lindenberg S, Ernst E et al (1999) DNA strand breaks in human spermatozoa: a possible factor to be considered in couples suffering from unexplained infertility. Acta Obstet Gynecol Scand 78:622–625
53. Saleh RA, Agarwal A, Nelson DR et al (2002) Increased sperm nuclear DNA damage in normozoospermic infertile men: a prospective study. Fertil Steril 78(2):313–318
54. Sergerie M, Laforest G, Bujan L et al (2005) Sperm DNA fragmentation: threshold value in male fertility. Hum Reprod 20(12):3446–3451
55. Seli E, Gardner DK, Schoolcraft WB et al (2004) Extent of nuclear DNA damage in ejaculated spermatozoa impacts on blastocyst development after in vitro fertilization. Fertil Steril 82:378–383
56. Borini A, Tarozzi N, Bizzaro D et al (2006) Sperm DNA fragmentation: paternal effect on early post-implantation embryo development in ART. Hum Reprod 21:2876–2881
57. Benchaib M, Lornage J, Mazoyer C et al (2007) Sperm deoxyribonucleic acid fragmentation as a prognostic indicator of assisted reproductive technology outcome. Fertil Steril 87:93–100
58. Pacey AA (2010) Environmental and lifestyle factors associated with sperm DNA damage. Hum Fertil (Camb) 13(4):189–193
59. Potts RJ, Newbury CJ, Smith G et al (1999) Sperm chromatin damage associated with male smoking. Mutat Res 423:103–111
60. Chatterjee R, Haines GA, Perera DM et al (2000) Testicular and sperm DNA damage after treatment with fludarabine for chronic lymphocytic leukaemia. Hum Reprod 15:762–766
61. Morris ID (2002) Sperm DNA damage and cancer treatment. Int J Androl 25:255–261
62. Chan D, Delbès G, Landry M et al (2012) Epigenetic alterations in sperm DNA associated with testicular cancer treatment. Toxicol Sci 125(2):532–543
63. Kumar D, Salian SR, Kalthur G et al (2013) Semen abnormalities, sperm DNA damage and global hypermethylation in health workers occupationally exposed to ionizing radiation. PLoS One 8(7):e69927. doi:10.1371/journal.pone.0069927
64. Cordelli E, Fresegna AM, Leter G et al (2003) Evaluation of DNA damage in different stages of mouse spermatogenesis after testicular X irradiation. Radiat Res 160(4):443–451
65. Kobayashi H, Larson K, Sharma RK et al (2001) DNA damage in patients with untreated cancer as measured by the sperm chromatin structure assay. Fertil Steril 75:469–475

66. Saleh RA, Agarwal A, Sharma RK et al (2003) Evaluation of nuclear DNA damage in spermatozoa from infertile men with varicocele. Fertil Steril 80:1431–1436
67. Nasr Esfahani MH, Tavalaee M (2012) Origin and role of DNA damage in varicocele. Int J Fertil Steril 6(3):141–146
68. Alvarez JG, Sharma RK, Ollero M et al (2002) Increased DNA damage in sperm from leukocytospermic semen samples as determined by the sperm chromatin structure assay. Fertil Steril 78:319–329
69. Erenpreiss J, Hlevicka S, Zalkalns J et al (2002) Effect of leukocytospermia on sperm DNA integrity: a negative effect in abnormal semen samples. J Androl 23:717–723
70. Das M, Al-Hathal N, San-Gabriel M et al (2013) High prevalence of isolated sperm DNA damage in infertile men with advanced paternal age. J Assist Reprod Genet 30(6):843–848
71. Singh NP, Muller CH, Berger RE (2003) Effects of age on DNA double-strand breaks and apoptosis in human sperm. Fertil Steril 80:1420–1430
72. García-Ferreyra J, Romero R, Hilario R et al (2012) High levels of DNA fragmentation observed in an infertile population attending a fertility center are related to advanced paternal age. Fert In Vitro 2:5. http://www.omicsgroup.org/journals/2165-7491/2165-7491-2-113.php?aid=9646%3Faid=9646
73. Sergerie M, Mieusset R, Croute F et al (2007) High risk of temporary alteration of semen parameters after recent acute febrile illness. Fertil Steril 88(4):970.e1–7
74. Potts JM, Pasqualotto FF (2003) Seminal oxidative stress in patients with chronic prostatitis. Andrologia 35(5):304–308
75. Kullisaar T, Türk S, Punab M et al (2008) Oxidative stress in leucocytospermic prostatitis patients: preliminary results. Andrologia 40(3):161–172
76. Hu YY, Cao SS, Lü JQ (2013) Impact of chronic prostatitis/chronic pelvic pain syndrome on sperm DNA fragmentation and nucleoprotein transition. Zhonghua Nan Ke Xue 19(10):907–911
77. Zhou JF, Xiao WQ, Zheng YC et al (2006) Increased oxidative stress and oxidative damage associated with chronic bacterial prostatitis. Asian J Androl 8(3):317–323
78. Henkel R, Maass G, Hajimohammad M et al (2003) Urogenital inflammation: changes of leucocytes and ROS. Andrologia 35(5):309–313
79. Sharma RK, Pasqualotto FF, Nelson DR et al (1999) The reactive oxygen species-total antioxidant capacity score is a new measure of oxidative stress to predict male infertility. Hum Reprod 14(11):2801–2807
80. Fraga GG, Motchnik PA, Shigenaga MK et al (1991) Ascorbic acid protects against endogenous oxidative DNA damage in human sperm. Proc Natl Acad Sci U S A 88:11003–11006
81. Sun JG, Jurisicova A, Casoer RF (1997) Detection of deoxyribonucleic acid fragmentation human sperm: correlation with fertilization in vitro. Biol Reprod 56:519–524
82. Murphy AB, Macejko A, Taylor A et al (2009) Chronic prostatitis: management strategies. Drugs 69(1):71–84
83. Krieger JN, Lee SW, Jeon J et al (2008) Epidemiology of prostatitis. Int J Antimicrob Agents 31(Suppl 1):S85–S90
84. Roberts RO, Jacobson DJ, Girman CJ et al (2002) Prevalence of prostatitis-like symptoms in a community based cohort of older men. J Urol 168(6):2467–2471
85. Nickel JC, Downey J, Hunter D et al (2001) Prevalence of prostatitis-like symptoms in a population based study using the National Institutes of Health chronic prostatitis symptom index. J Urol 165:842–845
86. Collins MM, Stafford RS, O'Leary MP et al (1998) How common is prostatitis? A national survey of physician visits. J Urol 159(4):1224–1228
87. Britton JJ, Carson CC (1998) Prostatitis. AUA Update Series 17:154–159
88. Schappert SM (1994) National Ambulatory Medical Care Survey: 1991 summary. Vital Health Stat 13(116):1–110
89. Riley DE, Krieger JN (2002) X Chromosomal short tandem repeat polymorphisms near the phosphoglycerate kinase gene in men with chronic prostatitis. Biochim Biophys Acta 1586(1):99–107

90. Dohle GR (2003) Inflammatory-associated obstructions of the male reproductive tract. Andrologia 35(5):321–324
91. El-Bayoumi MA, Hamada TA, El-Mokaddem HH (1982) Male infertility: etiologic factors in 385 consecutive cases. Andrologia 14(4):333–339
92. Li HJ, Xu P, Liu JS et al (2004) Prevalence of chronic prostatitis and its effects on male infertility. Zhonghua Yi Xue Za Zhi 84(5):369–371
93. Gorczyca W, Gong J, Darzynkiewicz Z (1993) Detection of DNA strand breaks in individual apoptotic cells by the in situ terminal deoxynucleotidyl transferase and nick translation assays. Cancer Res 53:1945–1951
94. Haines G, Marples B, Daniel P et al (1998) DNA damage in human and mouse spermatozoa after in vitro-irradiation assessed by the comet assay. Adv Exp Med Biol 444:79–91; discussion 92–93
95. Evenson DP, Darzynkiewicz Z, Melamed MR (1980) Relation of mammalian sperm chromatin heterogeneity to fertility. Science 210(4474):1131–1133
96. Muriel L, Garrido N, Fernández JL et al (2006) Value of the sperm deoxyribonucleic acid fragmentation level, as measured by the sperm chromatin dispersion test, in the outcome of in vitro fertilization and intracytoplasmic sperm injection. Fertil Steril 85(2):371–383
97. Zhang LH, Qiu Y, Wang KH et al (2010) Measurement of sperm DNA fragmentation using bright-field microscopy: comparison between sperm chromatin dispersion test and terminal uridine nick-end labeling assay. Fertil Steril 94(3):1027–1032
98. Ribas-Maynou J, García-Peiró A, Fernandez-Encinas A et al (2012) Double stranded sperm DNA breaks, measured by Comet assay, are associated with unexplained recurrent miscarriage in couples without a female factor. PLoS One 7(9):e44679. doi:10.1371/journal.pone.0044679
99. Evenson DP, Wixon R (2008) Data analysis of two in vivo fertility studies using Sperm Chromatin Structure Assay-derived DNA fragmentation index vs. pregnancy outcome. Fertil Steril 90(4):1229–1231
100. Dada R, Thilagavathi J, Venkatesh S et al (2011) Genetic testing in male infertility. Open Reprod Sci J 3:42–56
101. Sharma RK, Sabanegh E, Mahfouz R et al (2010) TUNEL as a test for sperm DNA damage in the evaluation of male infertility. Urology 76(6):1380–1386
102. Simon L, Lutton D, McManus J et al (2011) Sperm DNA damage measured by the alkaline Comet assay as an independent predictor of male infertility and in vitro fertilization success. Fertil Steril 95(2):652–657
103. Ribas-Maynou J, García-Peiró A, Fernández-Encinas A et al (2013) Comprehensive analysis of sperm DNA fragmentation by five different assays: TUNEL assay, SCSA, SCD test and alkaline and neutral Comet assay. Andrology 1(5):715–722
104. Zini A, San Gabriel M, Baazeem A (2009) Antioxidants and sperm DNA damage: a clinical perspective. J Assist Reprod Genet 26(8):427–432
105. Baker K, McGill J, Sharma R et al (2013) Pregnancy after varicocelectomy: impact of postoperative motility and DFI. Urology 81(4):760–766
106. Santos EP, López-Costa S, Chenlo P et al (2011) Impact of spontaneous smoking cessation on sperm quality: case report. Andrologia 43(6):431–435
107. Talevi R, Barbato V, Fiorentino I et al (2013) Protective effects of in vitro treatment with zinc, d-aspartate and coenzyme q10 on human sperm motility, lipid peroxidation and DNA fragmentation. Reprod Biol Endocrinol 11(1):81
108. Lewis SE, John Aitken R, Conner SJ et al (2013) The impact of sperm DNA damage in assisted conception and beyond: recent advances in diagnosis and treatment. Reprod Biomed Online 27(4):325–337
109. Greco E, Romano S, Iacobelli M et al (2005) ICSI in cases of sperm DNA damage: beneficial effect of oral antioxidant treatment. Hum Reprod 20(9):2590–2594

Testicular Pathology

Fulvio Colombo, Giorgio Gentile, and Alessandro Franceschelli

13.1 Cryptorchidism

Cryptorchidism is the commonest congenital anomaly affecting the genitalia of newborn male infants.

The cause may be related to an intrinsic testicular defect or lack of maternal gonadotropins. Approximately 10 % of instances are bilateral. The most common location is at the external inguinal ring [1].

The testes normally descend into the scrotum at 7 months' gestation. The incidence of cryptorchidism therefore decreases with age: it is 30 % in premature infants, 3 % in newborns, 1.5 % at 1 month and 0.75 % at 1 year of age [1].

Most recent data reported that at 1 year of age, nearly 1 % of all full-term male infants have cryptorchidism [2].

A patent processus vaginalis is present in 90 % of patients, while inguinal hernia in 25 % [1].

The most useful classification of cryptorchidism is clinical, distinguishing into *palpable* and *non-palpable* testes [3].

The clinical management is decided by the location and presence of the testes:

- In the presence of *palpable* and retractile testes, the clinical approach should be initially conservative.
- In case of bilateral *non-palpable* testes, an immediate endocrinological and genetic evaluation is necessary.

From the etiological point of view, we can distinguish two kinds of undescended testicle:

- Those in which the gubernaculum has gone "off course", and we call them *ectopic testes*.
- Those in which the descent to the bottom of the scrotum has been incomplete, but "on course". We call them "incompletely descended" or *dystopic testes*.

In case of *ectopic testicle*, it has to be searched into one of four possible locations:

- Inguinal, in the abdominal wall, near the external inguinal ring
- Perineal
- Penile, near the base of the shaft
- Crural, in the thigh

In case of *dystopic testicle*, it moves up and down and can be defined according to its range of movement as:

- Abdominal, when the testicle may move in and out of the internal inguinal ring
- Inguinal, when it moves along the inguinal canal
- Emergent, when it appears at the external ring
- High retractile, when it moves up and down but cannot be made to go to the bottom of the scrotum
- Low retractile, when it descends to the bottom of the scrotum only in particular conditions (warm bath, under general anaesthesia, hand traction)

Low retractile testes are essentially normal and will always end up in the scrotum with puberty [4].

Possible complications of undescended testis could be [4]:

- Torsion: a peritoneal sac is often associated with an undescended testicle, making it prone to torsion.
- Infertility: common only in case of bilateral undescended testicles, not with unilateral.
- Cancer: about one in ten testicular tumours is associated with undescended testicle.

13.1.1 Diagnosis

Physical examination is sufficient for differentiating between palpable and non-palpable testes. The groin region may be "milked" towards the scrotum to detect the possible attraction of the testis into the scrotum. A retractile testis can generally be brought into the scrotum until a cremasteric reflex will retract it into the groin again [5].

A unilateral, non-palpable testis and an enlarged contralateral testis suggest testicular absence or atrophy, but this should not avoid surgical exploration. An inguinal, non-palpable testis requires specific visual inspection of the femoral, penile and perineal regions in order to exclude an ectopic testis [3].

When no testicle can be felt on one side, it is often in the inguinal canal. The testicle is easily found with a computed tomography (CT) scan, even in the abdomen [4].

Diagnostic laparoscopy is the only examination that can reliably confirm or exclude an intra-abdominal, inguinal and absent/vanishing testis (non-palpable testis). Before carrying out laparoscopic assessment, examination under general anaesthesia is recommended because some, originally non-palpable, testes could be palpable under anaesthetic conditions [6].

13.1.2 Treatment

Although 90 % of testicles are in the scrotum at birth, the next 9 % do not descend until 12 months, after which no more do [4]. Treatment should be done as early as possible, around 1 year of age, starting after 6 months and finishing preferably at 12 months of age, or 18 months at the latest. The timing is driven by the final adult results on spermatogenesis and hormone production, as well as the risk for tumours [7, 8].

After puberty the chance of improving fertility is minimal, and the risk of cancer increases rapidly, but most young men wish to keep both testes. When an undescended testicle is found in a mature grown man, orchiectomy is the procedure that should be advised in view of the risks of malignancy [4].

13.1.2.1 Medical Therapy
Taking into account the hormonal dependence of testicular descent, the use of human chorionic gonadotrophin (hCG) or gonadotrophin-releasing hormone (GnRH) is recommended, with maximum success rates of 20 %. However, it must be considered that almost 20 % of descended testes have the risk of reascending later [3].

In addition, the price that the patient will have to pay will be a premature puberty, with stunting of growth from early fusion of epiphyses [4].

A total dose of 6,000–9,000 U hCG (depending on weight and age) is given in four doses over a period of 2–3 weeks, along with GnRH, given for 4 weeks as a nasal spray at a dose of 1.2 mg/day, divided into three doses per day [3].

Medical treatment may be beneficial before surgical intervention (orchidolysis and orchidopexy) or afterwards (low intermittent dosages), in terms of increasing the chances of fertility in later life [9].

13.1.2.2 Surgery

Palpable Testis
Surgery for a palpable testis includes orchidofunicololysis and orchidopexy, via an inguinal approach, with success rates of up to 92 %. It is important to remove and dissect all cremasteric fibres to prevent secondary retraction [3].

Through a crease incision over the internal ring, the external oblique is opened, and the testicle is mobilized, taking care not to injure its artery or the vas deferens. The testicular vessels are followed up behind the peritoneum and mobilized medially by dividing fibrous bands. This allows the testicle to be placed in a sac between the dartos muscle and skin of the scrotum, without tension [4].

Associated problems, such as an open processus vaginalis, must be carefully dissected and closed. There should be no fixation sutures or they should be made between the tunica vaginalis and the dartos muscle. The lymph drainage of a testis that has undergone surgery for orchidopexy has been changed from iliac drainage to iliac and inguinal drainage (this is important in the event of later malignancy).

Scrotal orchidopexy can be considered in less severe case and when performed by surgeons with experience using that approach [3].

Non-palpable Testis

Inguinal surgical exploration with possible laparoscopy should be attempted for non-palpable testes. There is a significant chance of finding the testis via an inguinal incision. In rare cases, it is necessary to search into the abdomen if there are no vessels or vas deferens in the groin. Laparoscopy is the best way of examining the abdomen for a testis. In addition, either removal or orchidolysis and orchidopexy can be performed via laparoscopic access [10].

For boys aged ≥10 years with an intra-abdominal testis, with a normal contralateral testis, removal is an option because of the theoretical risk of later malignancy. In pre-pubertal boys, an effort should be made to preserve the testis. The exact location of the testis should be provided by CT scan and confirmed by laparoscopy [4].

In bilateral intra-abdominal testes, or in boys younger than 10 years, a one-stage or two-stage Fowler-Stephens procedure can be performed. In the event of a two-stage procedure, the testicular vessels are laparoscopically clipped or coagulated proximally to the testis as a first step, to allow development of collateral vasculature [11].

Six months later, a second operation provides the mobilization of the testicle downwards into the scrotum, by which time it will have acquired a new blood supply from the artery to the vas and it is safe to divide the testicular vessels [4].

This second-stage procedure, in which the testis is brought directly over the symphysis and next to the bladder into the scrotum, can also be performed by laparoscopy. The testicular survival rate in the one-stage procedure varies between 50 and 60 %, with success rates increasing up to 90 % for the two-stage procedure. Microvascular autotransplantation can also be performed with a 90 % testicular survival rate. However, the procedure requires skilled and experienced surgeons [12].

Ectopic testes never find their way into the scrotum and require orchidopexy [4].

13.1.3 Prognosis

Although boys with one undescended testis have a lower fertility rate, they have the same paternity rate as those with bilateral descended testes. Boys with bilateral undescended testes have lower fertility and paternity rates.

Boys with an undescended testis have an increased risk of developing testicular malignancy. Screening both during and after puberty is therefore recommended for these boys [3].

Pre-pubertal orchidopexy may decrease the risk of testicular cancer, and early surgical intervention is indicated in children with cryptorchidism.

Boys with retractile testes do not need medical or surgical treatment, but require close follow-up until puberty [3].

13.2 Testicular Torsion

Testicular torsion is one of the most common emergencies in urology. It may occur at any age, but is most common around puberty [4]. About one-half of instances occur during sleep. Although the cause is unknown, poor fixation of the testis within the tunica vaginalis (the so-called bell clapper deformity) is most often given as the origin [1].

It results in twisting of the spermatic cord and occlusion of the venous or arterial supply to the testis. It is a true vascular emergency that, if not treated within 3–4 h after onset of pain, causes a complete infarction of the testis, followed by its atrophy [1].

Clinical presentation entails a sudden onset of pain and swelling in the testicle. Patients often recall attacks of pain that come on and are relieved equally suddenly (a history of such warning attacks is sufficient reason to explore the testicle and fix it). On examination, the scrotum is tender, red and swollen, and it is seldom possible to distinguish testis from the epididymis [4].

The first classification classically distinguishes two forms [4]:

- *Extravaginal* torsion, rarely seen in newborn boys, in which the testicle has rotated on the spermatic cord and it is almost never possible to save the testis by untwisting it
- *Intravaginal* torsion, in which the tunica vaginalis may be unusually roomy even with a normally descended testicle, and the testis and epididymis can twist on a stalk (like a light bulb in its socket)

The differential diagnosis is from [4]:

- Mumps orchitis, which never attacks boys before puberty
- Epididymitis, which is often secondary to urinary infections

- Fat necrosis, occasionally seen in infants
- Cancer, which in older boys and men can present with inflammation
- Torsion of an appendix testis, which is difficult to be distinguished from torsion of the testis without exploration
- Incarcerated inguinal hernia

13.2.1 Diagnosis

No investigation should be allowed to delay surgical exploration. A Doppler or radioisotope scan may show absence of arterial circulation in the testicle but is justified only if it will not delay matters [4].

Generally, no harm results from scrotal exploration if epididymitis is found, but much harm can result from delay in treating testicular torsion [1].

13.2.2 Treatment

It is important to untwist the testicle before it dies from ischaemia [4]; therefore, the treatment depends on the interval from onset of pain to presentation in the emergency room.

Within 4 h of onset, manual detorsion under local anaesthesia of the testicular cord should be attempted (the testes twist towards the midline as seen from the feet). If manual detorsion is successful, elective bilateral orchidopexy is indicated within the next few days. If it is not successful, immediate surgical exploration is indicated [1].

If presentation is between 4 and 24 h from pain onset, immediate surgical exploration, detorsion and bilateral orchidopexy should be performed [1].

If more than 24 h have passed since onset of pain, surgical exploration is indicated, but preservation of testicular function is doubtful [1].

In these cases, orchiectomy and placement of a testicular prosthesis is the treatment of choice.

The testicle is explored through a transverse scrotal incision. The tunica vaginalis is opened and the testicle is untwisted. If there is any doubt about the viability of the testis, it can be incised to see if it still bleeds. All too often it is necrotic and must be removed [4].

In case of *torsion of the appendix testis*, tiny cysts are usually present at the upper pole, one on the epididymis (Wolffian duct origin) and the other on the testis (Mullerian duct origin). Apart from being of interest to embryologists either can twist on its stalk, exactly mimicking torsion of the testicle and equally requiring urgent exploration [4].

Because torsion occurs in about 10 % of cases on the other side, the other testicle should be fixed then or at a later operation.

13.3 Testicular Microlithiasis

Testicular microlithiasis (TM) is a relatively uncommon condition characterized by the presence of multiple, 1-mm to 3-mm foci of increased echogenicity distributed randomly in the testicular parenchyma, detected incidentally during scrotal ultrasound (US). Its incidence varies according to different reports: in healthy men, the incidence ranges between 1.5 and 5.6 % and in subfertile population between 0.8 and 20.0 % [13–15], but it increases over 50 % in patients with testicular cancer [16–18].

TM usually affects both testes, but may be unilateral and can be focal or diffuse.

The exact aetiology of TM is unclear. It is suggested that these calcified concretions within the lumen of seminiferous tubules originate from sloughing of degenerated intratubular cells and failure of the Sertoli cells to phagocyte the debris [19].

TM has been associated with several urological diseases, including testicular cancer (TGCT), intratubular germ cell neoplasia (ITGCNU), cryptorchidism (testicular dysgenesis), varicocele, Klinefelter's syndrome, hypogonadism and infertility.

The relationship between TM and infertility is not well understood even if decreased fertility could be expected because the majority of seminiferous tubules can be obstructed by intratubular calcifications. Infertile patients with TM may have significant reductions in sperm migrations and motility. However, although some authors have reported abnormal semen parameters in infertile men with TM, others have found no significant difference among infertile men with or without TM with no significant differences in sperm count, motility or morphology in terms of sperm function between infertile men with or without TM [13, 14, 17].

The clinical importance of TM is not well clarified: because they can often be observed in association with germ cell tumours, many authors suggest to consider them as a possible "marker" of testicular cancer and to perform a prolonged scrotal ultrasound follow-up of these patients in order to recognize possible testicular tumours.

However, still today, the debate continues because many of the observations who link TM and testicular cancer are based on retrospective series [20, 21].

Many studies report in fact the co-association between testicular tumour and TM, but few ones describe the actual risk of development of a testicular cancer after TM [22, 23].

Serter et al. identified TM in 53 of 2,179 (2.4 %) asymptomatic men (age 17–42 years), but none had testicular tumour [24]. Similarly, Peterson et al. reported TM in 84 of 1,504 asymptomatic men (5.6 %) and 1 man without TM who had TGCT; they concluded that testicular microlithiasis is a common finding in asymptomatic men that may not be related to testicular cancer [15].

DeCastro et al. [23] screened 1,504 healthy men (age between 18 and 35 years) and detected 84 cases of TM (5.6 % prevalence). Even if at 5-year follow-up one man had developed a TGCT (64 months after initial screening), implying increased risk of developing testicular cancer compared with the general population, the authors concluded that most men with TM would have not developed a testicular cancer and that, for this reason, an intensive screening program for men with testicular microlithiasis is not cost-effective and would have done little to improve outcomes associated with testicular cancer [23].

Richenberg et al. performed a pooled analysis of literature data: a total of four patients (1 %; 95 % CI 0.4–2.6 %) among the 389 patients who were included in the study developed during the follow-up period a testicular cancer (median follow-up range 29–62 months).

Of these four patients, three had coexisting risk factors, one atrophied testis and two with previous history of testicular germ cell cancer. Excluding these patients from the final analysis, only one patient in 386 with TM and no coexisting risk factors developed cancer during follow-up (0.26 %; 95 % CI 0.05–1.45 %). They concluded that the literature reports a high association between testicular microlithiasis and testicular cancer, but that their meta-analysis did not suggest a causal link between microlithiasis and cancer. In the absence of additional risk factors, surveillance is not advocated, while in the presence of additional risk factors, surveillance with regular follow-up is recommended [25].

Recently Tan et al. [26] in their systematic review and meta-analysis summarized literature data about TM: management should depend on the clinical context. In healthy, asymptomatic individuals, the absolute risk of concurrent or interval TGCT or ITGCNU is very low. In patients who undergo scrotal ultrasound because of sub- or infertility, cryptorchidism or a personal history of germ cell tumour and for this reason already are at an elevated risk of testicular cancer, the presence of TM further increases the risk of a concurrent diagnosis of ITGCNU or germ cell tumours. In their pooled analysis, the estimated summary risk ratio was 8.5. However, even in the presence of risk factors, in contrast with other authors that recommend performing testicular biopsy [16], they suggest only to follow up these patients regularly.

13.4 Testicular Trauma

Testicular trauma most commonly occurs in young men between 15 and 40 years. Testicular trauma may be the consequence of blunt or penetrating trauma [27].

13.4.1 Blunt Trauma

Blunt trauma to the scrotum can be responsible for testicular dislocation, testicular haematocele and testicular rupture, associated or not to scrotal haematoma.

Testicular dislocation is quite rare; it is more common in motor vehicle accidents and in these cases can be also bilateral. Possible sites with relative frequency are superficial inguinal 50 %, pubic 18 %, penile 8 %, canalicular 8 %, truly abdominal 6 %, perineal 4 %, acetabular 4 % and crural 2 %.

Traumatic dislocation of the testicle is treated by manual replacement and secondary orchidopexy. If primary manual reposition cannot be performed, immediate orchidopexy is indicated [28].

Haematocele can be treated conservatively if it is smaller than three times the size of the contralateral testis [27]. Larger haematoceles or growing ones in fact can require delayed surgery, because conservative treatment often fails. Early surgical intervention resulted in preservation of the testis in more than 90 % of cases compared to delayed surgery, which resulted in orchiectomy in 45–55 % of patients [29–31].

Testicular fracture or rupture may occur because of a traumatic compression of the testis against the inferior pubic ramus or symphysis, resulting in a rupture of the tunica albuginea testis, haemorrhage and extrusion of testicular contents into the scrotal sac.

The scrotum appears tender, swollen and ecchymotic, and the testis itself may be difficult to palpate. Ultrasound images show an irregular testicular outline, intra- and/or extra-testicular haematoma and heterogeneous testicular echotexture, with focal hyperechoic or hypoechoic areas in the testicular parenchyma corresponding to areas of haemorrhage or infarction [32].

In case of suspected testicular rupture, surgical exploration, with evacuation of haematoma, debridement of necrotic tissue and closure of the tunica albuginea, is indicated [31, 32].

13.4.2 Penetrating Scrotal Trauma

Penetrating trauma is usually due to gunshot wounds and less commonly to stab wounds, animal attacks and self-mutilation.

Testicular fractures and ruptures from penetrating injury are managed in the same way as are fractures and ruptures from blunt injury, with conservative debridement of non-viable tissue. Depending on the extent of the injury, primary reconstruction of the testis and scrotum can usually be performed. In patients with spermatic cord injury and complete vascular transection, immediate surgical exploration is mandatory with microvascular reanastomosis when possible.

When conservative surgical treatment is not possible, orchiectomy is indicated [27, 31, 32].

13.5 Testicular Cancer

13.5.1 Introduction

Testicular cancer accounts for about 5 % of all urological tumours, with an estimated incidence of 3–10 new cases occurring per 100,000 males/per year in Western countries [33].

The recent widespread use of high-frequency ultrasonography (US) has led to an increasing number of incidentally detected small testicular masses [34] (STMs), defined as non-palpable and less than 25 mm in diameter, and intrascrotal masses,

Table 13.1 Pathologic classification of testicular tumours

Germ cell tumours	Sex cord/gonadal stromal tumours	Miscellaneous nonspecific stromal tumours
Intratubular germ cell neoplasia	Leydig cell tumour	Ovarian epithelial tumour
Seminoma	Malignant Leydig cell tumour	Tumour of the collecting duct and rete testis
Spermatocytic seminoma	Sertoli cell tumour	Benign tumour of nonspecific stroma
Embryonal carcinoma	Malignant Sertoli cell tumour	Malignant tumour of nonspecific stroma
Yolk sac tumour	Granulosa	
Choriocarcinoma	Thecoma/fibroma group	
Teratoma	Incompletely differentiated or mixed sex cord tumours	
Tumours with more than one histologic type	Gonadoblastoma	

and more than 70 % of patients are diagnosed with stage I disease [35]; the early diagnosis and the good response to extreme chemo- and radiotherapy give an excellent cure rate to all the typology of testicular tumours [33].

Testicular tumours can be classified into three categories: germ cell tumours (90–95 %), cord stromal tumours and miscellaneous tumours (Table 13.1) [36].

13.5.2 Diagnosis of Testicular Cancer

Preoperative diagnosis of testicular cancer is based on identification of testicular nodules with the straight palpation of the testis and the exploration of inguinal lymph nodes that could be enlarged. The second step is *ultrasound (US) of both testes* and additional US of the retroperitoneum to screen for extensive retroperitoneal metastasis.

Serum tumour markers, both before and 5–7 days after orchiectomy (AFP and hCG) and LDH, should be always assessed [37]. A total body CT scan should be always carried out for detection of metastasis and retroperitoneal, mediastinal and supraclavicular nodes assessment.

The final diagnosis of testicular tumours is completed with the pathologic examination of the mass after inguinal exploration and orchiectomy with en bloc excision of the testis, tunica albuginea and spermatic cord. Organ-sparing surgery can be performed in some cases such as bilateral tumour [38] or solitary testes or incidental detection of STMs with intraoperative frozen section examination (FSE) of the mass [39].

13.6 Testicular Cancer's Staging System TNM (Table 13.2) [37]

13.6.1 Guidelines for the Treatment of Testicular Cancer

13.6.1.1 Seminoma Stage I

The most recommended management option is surveillance, due to the low risk of recurrence rate (<6 %) [37]; radiotherapy is not recommended as adjuvant therapy. one cycle of carboplatin-based chemotherapy can be used as alternative to surveillance [40].

Table 13.2 Testicular Cancer's Staging System TNM [37]

pT	*Primary tumour*[a]
pTX	Primary tumour cannot be assessed
pT0	No evidence of primary tumour (eg, histologic scar in testis)
pTis	Intratubular germ cell neoplasia (testicular intraepithelial neoplasia)
pT1	Tumour limited to testis and epididymis without vascular/lymphatic invasion: tumour may invade tunica albuginea but not tunica vaginalis
pT2	Tumour limited to testis and epididymis with vascular/lymphatic invasion or tumour extending through tunica albuginea with involvement of tunica vaginalis
pT3	Tumour invades spermatic cord with or without vascular/lymphatic invasion
pT4	Tumour invades scrotum with or without vascular/lymphatic invasion
N – Regional lymph nodes clinical	
NX	Regional lymph nodes cannot be assessed
N0	No regional lymph node metastasis
N1	Metastasis with a lymph node mass ≤2 cm in greatest dimension or multiple lymph nodes; none >2 cm in greatest dimension
N2	Metastasis with a lymph node mass >2 cm but ≤5 cm in greatest dimension or multiple lymph nodes; any one mass >2 cm but ≤5 cm in greatest dimension
N3	Metastasis with a lymph node mass >5 cm in greatest dimension
pN – Pathologic regional lymph nodes	
pNX	Regional lymph nodes cannot be assessed
pN0	No regional lymph node metastasis
pN1	Metastasis with a lymph node mass ≤2 cm in greatest dimension and ≤5 positive nodes; none >2 cm in greatest dimension
pN2	Metastasis with a lymph node mass >2 cm but <5 cm in greatest dimension; or >5 nodes positive, none >5 cm; or evidence of extranodal extension of tumour
pN3	Metastasis with a lymph node mass >5 cm in greatest dimension

(continued)

Table 13.2 (continued)

M – Distant metastasis			
MX	Distant metastasis cannot be assessed		
M0	No distant metastasis		
M1	Distant metastasis		
M1a	Nonregional lymph node(s) or lung		
M1b	Other sites		
pM – Pathologic distant metastasis			
MX	Distant metastasis cannot be assessed		
M0	No distant metastasis		
M1	Distant metastasis		
M1a	Nonregional lymph node(s) or lung		
M1b	Other sites		
S – Serum tumour markers			
Sx	Serum markers studies not available or not performed		
S0	Serum marker study levels within normal limits		
	LDH, U/l	*hCG, mIU/ml*	*AFP, ng/ml*
S1	<1.5×N and	<5,000 and	<1,000
S2	1.5–10×N or	5,000–50,000 or	1,000–10,000
S3	>10×N or	>50,000 or	>10,000

LDH lactate dehydrogenase, *N* upper limit of normal for the LDH assay, *hCG* human gonadotrophin, *AFP* α-fetoprotein
[a]Except for pTis and pT4, where radical orchidectomy is not always necessary for classification purposes, the extent of the primary tumour is classified after radical orchidectomy; see pT. In other circumstances, TX is used if no radical orchidectomy has been performed

13.6.1.2 Non-seminomatous Germ Cell Tumour (NSGCT) Stage I

In this case the treatments depend on vascular invasion: in case of no vascular invasion (low risk of recurrence/metastasis), a long-term surveillance (at least 5 years) close follow-up is the recommended option [41]; an alternative adjuvant chemotherapy or nerve-sparing retroperitoneal lymph node dissection (RPLND) can be proposed; if RPLND shows nodal involvement, two courses of PEB (cisplatin, etoposide, bleomycin) chemotherapy are the best option.

In case of vascular invasion (pT2–pT4), the high risk of metastasis indicates chemotherapy with two courses of PEB [42] or an alternative surveillance or nerve-sparing RPLND [43] in patients not willing to undergo adjuvant chemotherapy.

If pathologic stage II is revealed at RPLND, further chemotherapy should be considered.

13.6.1.3 Metastatic Germ Cell Tumours GR

In case of low-volume NSGCT stage IIA/B with elevated markers, it should be treated with three or four cycles of PE; in case of tumours without marker elevation, chemotherapy can be performed after histologic analysis with RPLND or biopsy 6 weeks after orchiectomy [44].

In case of NSGCT > stage IIC, three or four courses of PEB are the primary treatment of choice according to prognosis grade [44].

If serum levels of tumour markers are normal or normalizing, surgical resection of residual masses after chemotherapy in NSGCT is indicated.

Seminoma IIA/B can be treated with radiotherapy; chemotherapy can be used as a salvage treatment with the same schedule as for the corresponding prognostic groups of NSGCT.

In seminoma stage CS IIB, chemotherapy ($4 \times EP$ or $3 \times PEB$, in good prognosis) is an alternative to radiotherapy.

Seminoma stage $\geq$ IIC should be treated with primary chemotherapy according to the same principles used for NSGCT [45].

13.6.2 Testicular Stromal Tumours

Testicular stromal tumours are rare (<10 % of all testicular tumours); among a wide array of benign and malignant lesions, Leydig cell tumours and Sertoli cell tumours are the most common [46].

13.6.3 Leydig Cell Tumours

Leydig cell tumours represent 1–3 % of adult testicular tumours and 3 % in childhood [46, 47]. Only 7–10 % of them are malignant; no malignant tumours have occurred in the pre-pubertal population [47].

The clinical presentation usually is characterized by a painless enlarged testis but very often the diagnosis is incidental in course of testicular US; it is very often accompanied by hormonal disorders (80 % of cases) [48]. Nowadays, the good outcome of Leydig cell tumours treated by partial orchiectomy is widely demonstrated [47–49, 50], but the diagnosis of Leydig cell tumours is possible only often pathologic analysis, for this reason intraoperative FSE is mandatory [47]. In case of malignancy, orchiectomy and RPLND are the best options [46].

13.6.4 Sertoli Cell Tumours

They are rarer than Leydig cell tumours, accounting for 1 % of all testis tumours; malignancy is found in 10 % of cases. Clinical presentation is similar to Leydig cell tumours, such as frequency of incidental diagnosis [46].

Even in this case organ-sparing surgery with intraoperative FSE is a good option of treatment, but in case of histologic signs of malignancy, orchiectomy and RPLND are the treatment of choice [49].

13.6.5 Conclusions

The most common testis tumours derive from germ cells; nowadays the development of diagnostic allows their detection in an early stage.

The treatment of choice is orchiectomy with excellent cure rates when it is performed in early stages.

In advanced stages a multidisciplinary therapeutic approach offers an acceptable survival rate. Follow-up schedules are mandatory to initial staging and treatment.

Testicular stromal tumours are rare and usually benign; they can be treated by organ-sparing surgery associated with intraoperative FSE. In case of malignancy, orchiectomy and RPLND are the treatment of choice.

References

Cryptorchidism

1. Krane MB, Siroki RJ, Fitzpatrick RV (1999). Clinical Urology. ISIS pubblications, Chicago (Ill.-USA)
2. Berkowitz GS, Lapinski RH, Dolgin SE et al (1993) Prevalence and natural history of cryptorchidism. Pediatrics 92(1):44–49
3. Tekgül S, Dogan HS, Hoebeke P et al. Guidelines on pediatric urology. http://www.uroweb.org/gls/pdf/23%20Paediatric%20Urology_LR%20March%2025th.pdf
4. Blandy J Kaisary A (2010) Lecture Notes: Urology. 6th Edition. Wiley-Blackwell, NY, U.S.A.
5. Rabinowitz R, Hulbert WC Jr (1997) Late presentation of cryptorchidism: the etiology of testicular re-ascent. J Urol 157(5):1892–1894
6. Cisek LJ, Peters CA, Atala A et al (1998) Current findings in diagnostic laparoscopic evaluation of the nonpalpable testis. J Urol 160(3 Pt 2):1145–1149; discussion 1150
7. Hadziselimovic F, Hocht B, Herzog B et al (2007) Infertility in cryptorchidism is linked to the stage of germ cell development at orchidopexy. Horm Res 68(1):46–52
8. Hadziselimovic F, Herzog B (2001) The importance of both an early orchidopexy and germ cell maturation for fertility. Lancet 358(9288):1156–1157
9. Schwentner C, Oswald J, Kreczy A et al (2005) Neoadjuvant gonadotropin releasing hormone therapy before surgery may improve the fertility index in undescended testes – a prospective randomized trial. J Urol 173(3):974–977
10. Jordan GH, Winslow BH (1994) Laparoscopic single stage and staged orchiopexy. J Urol 152(4):1249–1252
11. Bloom DA (1991) Two-step orchiopexy with pelviscopic clip ligation of the spermatic vessels. J Urol 145(5):1030–1033
12. Esposito C, Iacobelli S, Farina A et al (2010) Exploration of inguinal canal is mandatory in cases of non palpable testis if laparoscopy shows elements entering a closed inguinal ring. Eur J Pediatr Surg 20:138–139

Testicular Microlithiasis

13. von Eckardstein S, Tsakmakidis G, Kamischke A, Rolf C, Nieschlag E (2001) Sonographic testicular microlithiasis as an indicator of premalignant conditions in normal and infertile men. J Androl 22:818–824
14. de Gouveia Brazao CA, Pierik FH, Oosterhuis JW, Dohle GR, Looijenga LH, Weber RF (2004) Bilateral testicular microlithiasis predicts the presence of the precursor of testicular germ cell tumors in subfertile men. J Urol 171:158–160

15. Peterson AC, Bauman JM, Light DE, McMann LP, Costabile RA (2001) The prevalence of testicular microlithiasis in an asymptomatic population of men 18 to 35 years old. J Urol 166:2061–2064
16. van Casteren NJ, Looijenga LH, Dohle GR (2009) Testicular microlithiasis and carcinoma in situ overview and proposed clinical guideline. Int J Androl 32:279–287
17. Yee WS, Kim YS, Kim SJ, Choi JB, Kim SI, Ahn HS (2011) Testicular microlithiasis: prevalence and clinical significance in a population referred for scrotal ultrasonography. Korean J Urol 52(3):172–177
18. Richenberg J, Brejt N (2012) Testicular microlithiasis: is there a need for surveillance in the absence of other risk factors? Eur Radiol 22(11):2540–2546
19. Jungwirth A, Giwercman A, Tournaye H et al. (2012) European Association of Urology guidelines on Male Infertility: the 2012 update. Eur Urol. 62(2):324–332
20. Derogee M, Bevers RF, Prins HJ et al (2001) Testicular microlithiasis, a premalignant condition: prevalence, histopathologic findings, and relation to testicular tumor. Urology 57(6):1133–1137
21. Miller FN, Sidhu PS (2002) Does testicular microlithiasis matter? A review. Clin Radiol 57:883–890
22. Dagash H, Mackinnon EA (2007) Testicular microlithiasis: what does it mean clinically? BJU Int 99:157–160
23. DeCastro BJ, Peterson AC, Costabile RA (2008) A 5-year followup study of asymptomatic men with testicular microlithiasis. J Urol 179(4):1420–1423
24. Serter S, Gümüş B, Unlü M, Tunçyürek O, Tarhan S, Ayyildiz V, Pabuscu Y (2006) Prevalence of testicular microlithiasis in an asymptomatic population. Scand J Urol Nephrol 40:212–214
25. Richenberg J, Brejt N (2012) Testicular microlithiasis: is there a need for surveillance in the absence of other risk factors? Eur Radiol 22(11):2540–2546
26. Tan IB, Ang KK, Ching BC, Mohan C, Toh CK, Tan MH (2010) Testicular microlithiasis predicts concurrent testicular germ cell tumors and intratubular germ cell neoplasia of unclassified type in adults: a meta-analysis and systematic review. Cancer 116(19):4520–4523

Testicular Trauma

27. Summerton DJ, Kitrey ND, Lumen N, Serafetinidis E, Djakovic N (2012). EAU guidelines on iatrogenic trauma. Eur Urol 62(4):628–639
28. Schwartz SL, Faerber GJ (1994) Dislocation of the testes, as a delayed presentation of scrotal trauma. Urology 43:743
29. Cass AS, Luxenberg M (1991) Testicular injuries. Urology 37(6):528–530
30. Lee SH, Bak CW, Choi MH, Lee HS, Lee MS, Yoon SJ (2008) Trauma to male genital organs: a 10 year review of 156 patients, including 118 treated by surgery. BJU Int 101:211–215
31. Buckley JC, McAninch JW (2006) The diagnosis, management, and outcomes of pediatric renal injuries. Urol Clin North Am 33(1):33–40
32. Deurdulian C, Mittelstaedt CA, Chong WK, Fielding JR (2007) US of acute scrotal trauma: optimal technique, imaging findings, and management. Radiographics 27(2):357–369

Testicular Cancer

33. La Vecchia C, Bosetti C, Lucchini F et al (2010) Cancer mortality in Europe, 2000–2004, and an overview of trends since 1975. Ann Oncol 21(6):1323–1360
34. Steiner H, Holtl L, Maneschg C, Berger AP, Rogatsch H, Bartsch G, Hobisch A (2003) Frozen section analysis-guided organ-sparing approach in testicular tumors: technique, feasibility, and longterm results. Urology 62:508–513

35. Curado MP, Edwards B, Shin R et al (eds) (2007) Cancer incidence in five continents, vol 9, IARC Scientific Publications No. 160. International Association for Research on Cancer, Lyon
36. WHO histological classification of testis tumours (2004) In: Eble JN, Sauter G, Epstein JI, Sesterhenn IA (eds) Pathology and genetics. Tumours of the urinary system and male genital organs. IARC Press, Lyon, pp 250–262
37. Albers P, Albrecht W, Algaba F, Bokemeyer C, Cohn-Cedermark G, Fizazi K, Horwich A, Laguna MP, European Association of Urology (2011) EAU guidelines on testicular cancer: 2011 update. Eur Urol 60(2):304–319
38. Giannarini G, Dieckmann KP, Albers P et al (2010) Organ-sparing surgery for adult testicular tumours: a systematic review of the literature. Eur Urol 57:780–790
39. Gentile G, Brunocilla E, Franceschelli A et al (2013) Can testis-sparing surgery for small testicular masses be considered a valid alternative to radical orchiectomy? A prospective single centre study. Clin Genitourin Cancer 11:522–526
40. Schoffski P, Hohn N, Kowalski R et al (2007) Health-related quality of life (QoL) in patients with seminoma stage I treated with either adjuvant radiotherapy (RT) or two cycles of carboplatinum chemotherapy (CT): results of a randomized phase III trial of the German Interdisciplinary Working Party on Testicular Cancer. ASCO Annual Meeting Proceedings. Part 1. J Clin Oncol 25(Suppl 18S):5050
41. Oliver RT, Ong J, Shamash J et al (2004) Long-term follow-up of Anglian Germ Cell Cancer Group surveillance versus patients with stage 1 nonseminoma treated with adjuvant chemotherapy. Urology 63:556–561
42. Tandstad T, Dahl O, Cohn-Cedermark G et al (2009) Risk-adapted treatment in clinical stage I nonseminomatous germ cell testicular cancer: the SWENOTECA management program. J Clin Oncol 27:2122–2128
43. Donohue JP, Thornhill JA, Foster RS et al (1995) Clinical stage B nonseminomatous germ cell testis cancer: the Indiana University experience (1965–1989) using routine primary retroperitoneal lymph node dissection. Eur J Cancer 31A:1599–1604
44. International Germ Cell Cancer Collaborative Group (1997) International Germ Cell Consensus Classification: a prognostic factor-based staging system for metastatic germ cell cancers. J Clin Oncol 15:594–603
45. Krege S, Beyer J, Souchon R et al (2008) European consensus conference on diagnosis and treatment of germ cell cancer: a report of the second meeting of the European Germ Cell Cancer Consensus group (EGCCCG): part I. Eur Urol 53:478–496
46. Risk MC, Porter CR (2009) Management of non-germinal testicular tumors. World J Urol 27:507–512
47. Thomas JC, Ross JH, Kay R (2001) Stromal testis tumors in children: a report from the prepubertal testis tumor registry. J Urol 166:2338–2340
48. Carmignani L, Colombo R, Gadda F et al (2007) Conservative surgical therapy for Leydig cell tumor. J Urol 178:507–511
49. Brunocilla E, Gentile G, Schiavina R et al (2013) Testis-sparing surgery for the conservative management of small testicular masses: an update. Anticancer Res 33(11):5205–5210
50. Bozzini G, Rubino B, Maruccia S et al (2014) Role of frozen section examination in the management of testicular nodules: a useful procedure to identify benign lesions. Urol J. 2014;11(3):1687–1691

Endocrine Infertility

Giorgio D. Piubello

14.1 Definition

This chapter encompasses all spermatogenesis-altering conditions affecting the normal male endocrine balance. Such conditions can be caused by either testicular abnormalities (or other endocrine gland or pituitary-hypothalamus disorders) or the effect of exogenous substances (endocrine disruptors).

14.2 Epidemiology

Male infertility is caused by endocrine alterations in 18–30 % of cases [1].

14.3 Etiopathogenesis

14.3.1 Hypogonadisms

The development, endocrine function, and reproductive function of the gonads are regulated by the hypothalamic-pituitary-gonadal axis. In the hypothalamus, specialized neurons release pulses of gonadotropin-releasing hormone (GnRH), which modulates the secretion of gonadotropins from the pituitary gland. In turn, the anterior pituitary gland produces luteinizing hormone (LH) and follicle-stimulating hormone (FSH), which stimulate steroid secretion and germ cell production in the testes. A complex interaction of endogenous inputs, chronobiological signals, and exogenous stressors regulates the whole process.

G.D. Piubello
Istituto Medicina Interna D, Università degli Studi di Verona,
Piazzale L. A. Scuro 1, Verona 37134, Italy
e-mail: giorgiopiubello@alice.it

Table 14.1 Classification of male hypogonadism

Secondary hypogonadism (hypogonadism hypogonadotropic)
Panhypopituitarism
Failure of the gonadotrophic function of the pituitary
Isolated LH deficiency
Isolated FSH deficiency
Altered LH biological activity
Altered FSH biological activity
Primary hypogonadism (hypogonadism hypergonadotropic)
Congenital or acquired anorchidism
Cryptorchidism
Mumps orchitis
Genetic and developmental conditions: Klinefelter syndrome, androgen receptor, LH receptor and enzyme defects
Sertoli cell only syndrome
Radiation treatment or chemotherapy
Testicular trauma
Testicular torsion

Male hypogonadism is defined as a clinical situation presenting a deficit in the testicular function. This defect can be a consequence of a disorder first originating in the testis (primitive or hypergonadotropic hypogonadism) or can be caused by insufficient stimulation of pituitary gonadotropins in the testis (hypogonadotropic hypogonadism). This condition can in turn be due to a defect in the pituitary (secondary hypogonadotropic hypogonadism) or an alteration in the secretion of hypothalamic GnRH (tertiary hypogonadotropic hypogonadism). The classification of male hypogonadism is reported in Table 14.1.

Late-onset hypogonadism, a condition in which androgens decline with advancing age, is instead imputable to the hypothalamus-pituitary and/or the testes.

Isolated deficiencies of FSH and LH also have been reported. Subjects with the rare isolated LH deficiency show eunuchoid body habitus, large testes, and small-volume ejaculates containing few spermatozoa. Plasma testosterone is low while FSH levels are normal.

Isolated FSH deficiency is also a rare condition that allows normal virilization and testosterone levels, albeit with low levels of FSH and oligospermia or azoospermia. Its cause may be an FSH β-subunit deficiency, an idiopathic genetic defect, or excess inhibin-B (idiopathic or resulting from a granulosa cell tumor).

14.3.2 Testicular Steroidogenesis Congenital Disorders

Hormone biosynthesis is carried out in both the adrenal cortex and the gonads. Many steps of this process are common to both, while others are only possible in the adrenal cortex. A congenital deficit of an enzyme of one of the steps of steroidogenesis produces a deficit in the hormones of the next step, and an increase in the hormones of preceding steps.

A series of complex syndromes are produced by the lack of certain hormones, which should have been synthesized, and by the increase of their precursors in circulation.

The most common condition is reduced virilization in the male embryo (male pseudohermaphroditism). There are eight known enzymatic defects able to affect testosterone synthesis, the most frequent of which is 21-hydroxylase deficit, which accounts for 95 % of such defects.

14.3.3 Androgen Resistance Syndromes

Androgen resistance syndromes are caused by alterations of the androgen receptor or the 5α-reductase enzyme, which hinder the androgenic action. Virilization defects shown by affected individuals are highly variable and have been classified according to five phenotypic variants, ranging from complete testicular feminization syndrome to simple, and sometimes slight, virilization defects. Spermatogenesis is absent or reduced, but can be normal in rare cases.

14.3.4 Other Endocrine Diseases

14.3.4.1 Hyperprolactinemia

A chronic prolactin excess interferes with gonadic function, reducing testosterone levels and causing oligospermia. The mechanisms by which hyperprolactinemia inhibit testicular function are not yet fully verified, even though experimental data indicate that it is likely the result of a combined action at the pituitary-hypothalamic level (by reducing the GnRH/gonadotropic secretion) and at the testicular level (by interfering with testosterone synthesis and secretion). Spermatogenesis alterations are probably secondary with respect to the testosterone deficit, while it is unknown whether prolactin is able to act negatively at a tubular level.

A routine check of prolactin levels in asymptomatic infertile men is not recommended. In fact, mild increases in prolactin are of doubtful significance, as they may be caused by medications or several other medical conditions. Prolactin-secreting tumors are rare, with prolactin levels beyond 50 ng/mL appearing in adenomas larger than 1 cm [2].

14.3.4.2 Thyroid Disease

Male infertility is more frequent in thyroid diseases, particularly in hyperthyroidism [3, 4]. Nonetheless, most men with thyroid abnormalities are not infertile, either before or after treatment. Thyroid abnormalities, if present, often lead to oligospermia rather than azoospermia. The following mechanisms have been proposed: alterations in sex steroid metabolism, testicular and pituitary developmental abnormalities, changes in sex hormone binding globulin (SHBG), and increased levels of estradiol. Severe congenital hypothyroidism may cause global developmental abnormalities of the hypothalamic-pituitary-gonadal axis.

14.3.4.3 Growth Hormone Alterations

There are few data confirming a role of growth hormone (GH) in endocrine dysfunction in fertility [5]. In fact it is difficult to identify a reliable method of measuring GH secretion patterns that may relate to fertility. However, acromegaly may inhibit spermatogenesis [6].

14.3.4.4 Hyperestrogenism

High levels of estrogens caused by peripheral aromatization in adipose tissue, mainly in obese subjects, can inhibit pituitary function [7] and, therefore, spermatogenesis.

14.3.4.5 Cushing Syndrome

In Cushing syndrome, the glucocorticoid excess not only can suppress LH function but may also have a direct contributing role in affecting spermatogenesis and maturation arrest [8].

14.3.4.6 Diabetes Mellitus

Infertility rates in individuals with diabetes are higher than average (16 and 19.1 %, respectively, for primary and secondary infertility) [9]. Excessive weight, and obesity in particular, seem to be the leading contributors to infertility.

Three main dysfunctional mechanisms may be postulated to explain the sperm damage observed in diabetic patients: endocrine disorders, diabetic neuropathy, and oxidative stress. In insulin-dependent diabetes:

1. Leydig cell function and testosterone production decrease because of the lack of stimulatory effect of insulin on these cells
2. An insulin-dependent decrease in FSH reduces LH levels
3. The FSH decrease also reduces sperm output and fertility

As a result, in diabetic patients serum testosterone is decreased and gonadotropin levels are increased. Moreover, a steroidogenetic defect in Leydig cells can be observed.

14.3.5 Endocrine Disruptors

Endocrine manipulation in male infertility starts with ruling out possible endocrine disruptors [10].

Micropollutants in the environment, in particular steroid mimetics (in water supplies, food sources, etc.), may contribute to an overall decline in male fertility.

The increasing use of phytoestrogen has also been claimed to contribute. In fact, many dietary supplements contain significant levels of plant phytoestrogens that mimic testosterone and estrogen.

14.4 Diagnosis

Clinical history and physical examination are the cornerstones of the diagnosis: penis and testis volume, weight, height, and secondary sexual characteristics should be evaluated. The occurrence of headaches, visual disturbances, bitemporal visual field losses, cranial nerve palsies, and cerebrospinal fluid rhinorrhea should also be investigated.

A small set of basal hormones (testosterone, LH, FSH, estradiol, SHBG, prolactin) is usually sufficient for diagnosis (Fig. 14.1) [11]. It should be remembered that FSH and LH are secreted in short pulses, and a single measurement may not be sufficient to clarify the diagnosis.

14.4.1 Dynamic Tests

Persistent borderline low hormonal values may be further evaluated with the GnRH stimulation test, the clomiphene stimulation test, and the human chorionic gonadotropin (hCG) stimulation test [12].

14.4.1.1 GnRH Stimulation Test
This test is indicated in adult men with low testosterone levels and normal or low-to-normal gonadotropins. The patient receives GnRH 100 μg intravenously. LH and FSH both are expected to rise, with a peak occurring between 15 and 60 min; LH increases threefold to sixfold while FSH increases about 20–50 % above the baseline.

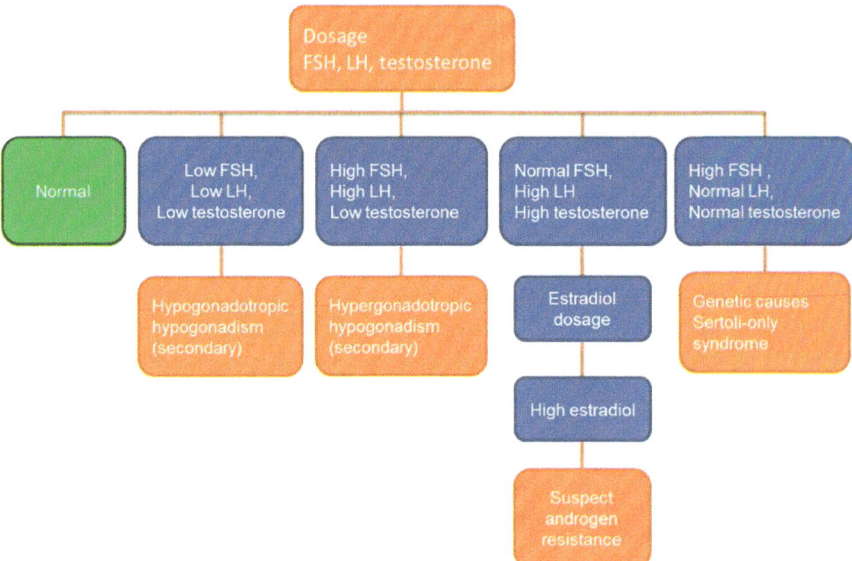

Fig. 14.1 Diagnostic flow chart of male hypogonadism

14.4.1.2 Clomiphene Stimulation Test

This test is indicated in suspected gonadotropin deficiencies. Clomiphene acts as an antiestrogen centrally and as a weak estrogen peripherally. The central antiestrogen effect, interrupting the negative feedback of estrogen on GnRH release, induces a rise in LH and FSH. The patient is treated for 5–7 days with 100 mg clomiphene citrate. A doubling of LH and a 20–50 % increase in FSH are considered normal.

14.4.1.3 Human Chorionic Gonadotropin Stimulation Test

The hCG stimulation test is indicated in adults, in the differential diagnosis of combined testicular and pituitary failure versus secondary hypogonadism. A single dose of hCG (5,000 IU intramuscularly) is administered, and testosterone values are measured at the baseline and every 24 h up to day 5. In adult hypogonadism the lack of an increase in testosterone after hCG suggests a lack of functioning testicular tissue. Conversely, a rise suggests an intact Leydig cell system. In gonadotropin deficiency with no primary testicular abnormality, the basal testosterone value should triple after hCG.

14.5 Therapy

Several sites can be influenced by selective drugs (Fig. 14.2).

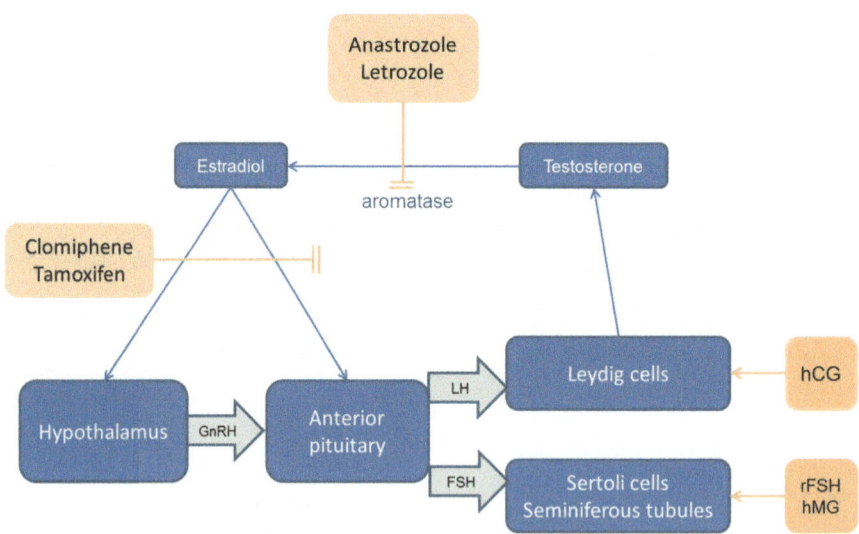

Fig. 14.2 Sites of action of drugs used for treating male hypogonadic infertility

14.5.1 Estrogen Receptor Modifiers

Both clomiphene and tamoxifen are selective estrogen receptor modifiers (SERMs); inhibiting estrogen receptor at the level of the pituitary, both FSH and LH levels increase. As a result testosterone increases, thus favoring sperm growth and maturation [13].

In hypogonadism and oligospermia, clomiphene is used as monotherapy [14]. Starting dose is 25 mg once daily; as clomiphene is normally available in 50-mg tablets, a starting dose might be 50 mg every other day. When testosterone remains low, clomiphene can be titrated up to 100 mg once daily.

Clomiphene has also been used on hypogonadic patients with azoospermia. Increases in testosterone in the testis may favor production of sufficient sperm in the ejaculate. Tamoxifen is used for the same indications [15], at a dosage of 10 mg once daily.

14.5.2 Aromatase Inhibitors

Anastrazole and letrozole are aromatase inhibitors, directly limiting estrogen feedback to the pituitary, thus increasing the production of FSH and LH [16]. Some men with severely defective sperm production have excessive aromatase activity, documented by low serum testosterone and relatively high estradiol levels. Aromatase inhibitors can increase endogenous testosterone production and serum testosterone levels. Treatment of infertile males with aromatase inhibitors has been associated with increased sperm production and return of sperm to the ejaculate in men with nonobstructive azoospermia.

Anastrazole (1 mg once daily) and letrozole (2.5 mg once daily) are used for impaired spermatogenesis, although this represents an off-label use.

Enclomiphene citrate [17] (an isomer of clomiphene) is in phase 3 trials for the treatment of hypogonadism infertility.

14.5.3 Gonadotropins

SERMs and aromatase inhibitors are effective and relatively inexpensive, and thus are used as first-line agents for the treatment of endocrine dysfunction in the hypogonadal infertile male.

However, in cases of severe hypogonadotropic hypogonadism, the LH homologue hCG is the gold standard for treatment [18]. hCG 2,000 IU subcutaneously, three times per week, is usually sufficient to achieve desired testosterone levels and induce spermatogenesis. Direct testosterone administration has proved to be ineffective [19, 20].

In congenital forms, a 6-month titration is often required to be followed by the use of recombinant FSH or an FSH analogue, human menopausal gonadotropin.

The usual dosage for both is 75 IU or 150 IU three times weekly, as the usual vial contains 75 IU. Even in acquired hypogonadotropic hypogonadism, however, combination hCG/FSH analogues may be more effective than hCG alone in stimulating spermatogenesis.

14.5.4 Future Therapy

The new horizon of idiopathic male infertility treatment is personalized pharmacogenetic therapy.

Gene therapy is one of the frontiers of modern medicine. A viral vector can be used as a delivery device to reconstitute a key missing promoter sequence encoding a vital protein for cellular function. Unfortunately, little is known about the genetic loci involved in spermatogenesis. Moreover, it may be difficult to affect testis and/or spermatozoa with gene therapy without affecting the germline. The Sertoli cells, because of their special tolerogenic properties, may represent an ideal candidate for cell-based gene therapy.

Further possibilities are tissue grafting and spermatogonial stem cell transplantation.

References

1. Isaia GC, Di Stefano M, Borin F, Gola D, Sciolla A (1997) Inquadramento clinico dell'ipogonadismo maschile. In: Molinatti GM, Fontana D (eds) Andrologia. Fisiopatologia e clinica. Verducci Editore, Roma, pp 157–166
2. Carter JN, Tyson JE, Tolis G, Van Vliet S, Faiman C, Friesen HG (1978) Prolactin secreting tumours and hypogonadism. N Engl J Med 299:847–852
3. Rajender S, Monica MG, Walter L, Agarwal A (2011) Thyroid, spermatogenesis, and male infertility. Front Biosci 3:843–855
4. Krassas GE, Poppe K, Glinoer D (2010) Thyroid function and human reproductive health. Endocr Rev 31:702–755
5. Shoham Z, Zalel Y, Jacobs HS et al (1994) The role of growth hormone in male infertility. Clin Endocrinol 41:1–5
6. Auger J, Kunstmann JM, Czyglik F et al (1995) Decline in semen quality among fertile men in Paris during the past 20 years. N Engl J Med 332:281–285
7. Michalakis K, Mintziori G, Kaprara A, Tarlatzis BC, Goulis DG (2013) The complex interaction between obesity, metabolic syndrome and reproductive axis: a narrative review. Metabolism 62:457–478
8. Gabrilove JL, Nicolis GL, Sohval AR (1974) The testis in Cushing's syndrome. J Urol 112:95–99
9. La Vignera S, Condorelli R, Vicari E, D'Agata R, Calogero AE (2012) Diabetes mellitus and sperm parameters. J Androl 33:145–153
10. Knez J (2013) Endocrine-disrupting chemicals and male reproductive health. Reprod Biomed Online 26:440–448
11. Sussman EM, Chudnovsky A, Niederberger CS (2008) Hormonal evaluation of the infertile male: has it evolved? Urol Clin North Am 35:147–155
12. Isidori AM, Giannetta E, Lenzi A (2008) Male hypogonadism. Pituitary 11:171–180

13. Chua ME, Escusa KG, Luna S, Tapia LC, Dofitas B, Morales M (2013) Revisiting oestrogen antagonists (clomiphene or tamoxifen) as medical empiric therapy for idiopathic male infertility: a meta-analysis. Andrology 1:749–757
14. Roth LW, Ryan AR, Meacham RB (2013) Clomiphene citrate in the management of male infertility. Semin Reprod Med 31:245–250
15. Moein MR, Tabibnejad N, Ghasemzadeh J (2012) Beneficial effect of tamoxifen on sperm recovery in infertile men with nonobstructive azoospermia. Andrologia 44(Suppl 1):194–198
16. Schlegel PN (2012) Aromatase inhibitors for male infertility. Fertil Steril 98:1359–1362
17. Kaminetsky J, Werner M, Fontenot G, Wiehle RD (2013) Oral enclomiphene citrate stimulates the endogenous production of testosterone and sperm counts in men with low testosterone: comparison with testosterone gel. J Sex Med 10:1628–1635
18. Paradisi R, Natali F, Fabbri R, Battaglia C, Seracchioli R, Venturoli S (2013) Evidence for a stimulatory role of high doses of recombinant human follicle-stimulating hormone in the treatment of male-factor infertility. Andrologia. doi:10.1111/and.12194
19. World Health Organization Task Force on the Diagnosis and Treatment of Infertility (1989) Mesterolone and idiopathic male infertility: a double-blind study. Int J Androl 12:254–264
20. Comhaire F (1990) Treatment of idiopathic testicular failure with high-dose testosterone undecanoate: a double-blind pilot study. Fertil Steril 54:689–693

Iatrogenic Infertility

15

Giovanni Beretta

15.1 Introduction

There are surgical treatments and a number of chemotherapeutic agents and drugs commonly used in therapies that may cause male infertility [1]. When the dispermia is due to medical or surgical causes, it is called iatrogenic infertility [2]. While reviews of iatrogenic causes of infertility in Western Europe reveal that these contribute to approximately 5 % of infertility both in men and women, in Africa this rate is higher [3].

15.2 Chemotherapeutic Drugs

The use of chemotherapeutic drugs in the treatment of cancer and in the management of autoimmune disease can interfere with fertility.

The *alkylating chemotherapy* agent group does the most damage to fertility. These drugs include cyclophosphamide (Cytoxan), chlorambucil (Leukeran), busulfan (Myleran), procarbazine (Natulan, Matulane), nitrosoureas (Carmustine, Lomustine), nitrogen mustard (Mustargen), and L-phenylalanine mustard (Alkeran). In high doses, platinum-based chemotherapy agents (cisplatin, oxaliplatin) or drugs like bleomycin (Blenoxane), often used to treat testicular cancer, can also damage fertility.

G. Beretta
Andrological and Reproductive Medicine Unit, Centro Demetra,
via Della Fortezza 6, Firenze 50129, Italy
e-mail: giovanniberetta@libero.it

© Springer International Publishing Switzerland 2015
G. Cavallini, G. Beretta (eds.), *Clinical Management of Male Infertility*,
DOI 10.1007/978-3-319-08503-6_15

15.2.1 Cyclophosphamide

Cyclophosphamide is one of the most frequently prescribed chemotherapeutic drugs. It is an anticancer and immunosuppressive agent commonly used in men of reproductive age and, when used in high dose or in combination regimens, can cause severe germ cell damage [4]. The damage done to spermatogenesis by cyclophosphamide appears to be dose dependent. A daily dose of 3.7 mg/kg body weight will produce oligospermia or even azoospermia, and this change is frequently permanent. Cyclophosphamide can also interfere with Leydig cell function, resulting in a reduced secretion of testosterone, thus increasing problems relating to infertility [5].

15.2.2 Chlorambucil

This is an aromatic nitrogen mustard that also acts as an alkylating agent. It is used in the treatments of lymphomas as well as in the management of leukemia. It can interfere with spermatogenesis, and its use frequently leads to azoospermia. Recovery in terms of fertility is very variable.

In the management of various types of cancer, it is common to use several different anticancer drugs in combination so that the effect upon the cancer is maximal. All these combinations will always give unpredictable and very uncertain recovery rate in terms of infertility [5] (Table 15.1).

It is very important to suggest patients to cryopreserve their semen before any chemotherapeutic treatment to save potential future fertility, as spermatogenesis will only return to normal in no more than 50 % of patients treated [6]. Certain cancers can cause men to have poor sperm quality, even prior to treatment [7, 8]. It is estimated that about 40 % of men with Hodgkin's disease and 50 % of those with testicular cancer will have low sperm counts at the time of diagnosis [9, 10]. This does not mean that these men should not consider sperm banking, as advances in reproductive techniques have made even poor-quality specimens useful for reproduction [11, 12].

15.3 Common Drugs That Can Cause Male Infertility

There are numerous drugs and medications that have been shown to have adverse effects on male fertility, acting through diverse mechanisms [2].

The mechanisms of impaired fertility include direct effects on germ cells or their supporting cells, on the delicately balanced HPG axis, on erectile or ejaculatory function, and on libido.

In a thorough fertility evaluation of the male partner, the physician should determine what medication the patient is taking and his social habits involving alcohol consumption, tobacco, and recreational drug use. Simply discontinuing the offending agents can reverse most adverse effects from drugs and medications.

Table 15.1 List of the drugs that can cause male infertility

Chemotherapy (dose to cause effect)	Known effect on sperm count
Chlorambucil (1.4 g/m^2)	Prolonged or permanent azoospermia
Cyclophosphamide (19 g/m^2)	
Procarbazine (4 g/m^2)	
Melphalan (140 mg/m^2)	
Cisplatin (500 mg/m^2)	
BCNU (1 g/m^2)	Azoospermia in adulthood if treated before puberty
CCNU (500 mg/m^2)	
Busulfan (600 mg/m^2)	Azoospermia likely, and they are often given with other highly sterilizing agents, adding to the effect
Ifosfamide (42 g/m^2)	
BCNU (300 mg/m^2)	
Nitrogen mustard	
Actinomycin D	
Doxorubicin (770 mg/m^2)	When used alone, cause only temporary reductions in sperm count. In conjunction with above agents, may be additive in causing azoospermia
Thiotepa (400 mg/m^2)	
Cytarabine (1 g/m^2)	
Vinblastine (50 g/m^2)	
Vincristine (8 g/m^2)	
Amsacrine	When used in conventional regimens, cause only temporary reductions in sperm count. In conjunction with above agents, may be additive in causing azoospermia
Bleomycin	
Dacarbazine	
Daunorubicin	
Epirubicin	
Etoposide	
Fludarabine	
Fluorouracil	
6-mercaptopurine	
Methotrexate	
Mitoxantrone	
Thioguanine	

Adapted from Devita et al. [5]

15.3.1 Nitrofurantoin

Nitrofurantoin has been shown to reduce the sperm count in animals and humans. This suppression is short and never permanent after the cessation of treatment.

15.3.2 Cimetidine

Cimetidine is an H2 inhibitor commonly used in the treatment of dyspepsia. It binds to the androgen receptors interfering with sperm production. Its action is short lived and reversible [2].

15.3.3 Sulfasalazine (Salazopyrin)

This drug is still widely used for the therapy of various different inflammatory bowel disorders, especially for ulcerative colitis. It causes a reduction of concentration and motility of the sperms and also alters the shape of sperm head. Upon cessation of therapy, the sperm count and motility will returns to normal [2].

15.3.4 Sex Steroids

Estrogens and testosterone will reduce gonadotropin secretion, and thus, therapy with testosterone will rapidly lead to azoospermia.

15.3.5 Gonadotropin-Releasing Hormone Analogs and Antiandrogens

These drugs, especially in the depot form, are frequently used in the treatment of hormone-dependent prostate cancer. These drugs quickly lead to azoospermia. Antiandrogens block the action of testosterone and can cause erectile failure. As prostate cancer is becoming more common and occurring in younger men, these aspects must be seriously considered [13–15].

15.4 Radiation Therapy

After World War II, with the use of atomic energy and the following incidental irradiation of men, it became clear that sperm production could be reduced to zero due to the effects of irradiation. In 1964, McLeod reported that the accidental exposure of men to radiation after an accident at the Oakridge Nuclear Plant caused azoospermia in more than half of them [16]. Radiation has its most potent effect upon spermatogonia, the type B spermatogonia being the most sensitive.

Radiation therapy can slow down or stop sperm cell production if the testicle is in or near the target area for the radiation. A lead shield can help protect the testicles, but radiation "scatters" within the body, so it is impossible to shield the testicles completely.

The likelihood of infertility after radiation depends on the dose to the testes, shielding, and fractionation (single dose vs. multiple doses). Doses as small as 0.1 Gy can result in decreased sperm counts, and doses of 1.5–4 Gy can result in permanent sterility. As previously noted, the Leydig cells (responsible for testosterone production) are less sensitive to the effects of radiation, with damage occurring at 30 Gy in mature males (20 Gy in prepubescent males).

If the testicles are not the primary radiation targets, shielding can be used. This technique protects the testicle(s) from receiving radiation. Fractionation is the technique of dividing the total dose of radiation into multiple smaller doses. For most side effects, fractionation is used to lessen their severity, but in this case fractionation (multiple smaller doses) causes more damage to sperm than a larger, single radiation dose.

Total body irradiation (TBI) is a technique used for preparation for stem cell and bone marrow transplants. As the name implies, it is irradiation of the entire body. It is estimated that 80 % of men who undergo TBI will have permanent azoospermia.

For those without permanent azoospermia, sperm counts are at their lowest 4–6 months after treatment. Counts typically return to their pretreatment levels 10–24 months after treatment but can take longer in those who received higher doses.

Radiation damage to the part of the brain that controls hormone production can sometimes interfere with the hormone messages that control sperm production [6].

15.5 Surgery

If the cancer surgery requires the removal of both testes, fertility is affected because of the inability to produce sperm [17, 18].

Surgery on the prostate, bladder, urethra, or colon can result in a condition called retrograde ejaculation.

In normal ejaculation, the semen is propelled through the urethra and the opening to the bladder closes off, allowing the semen to exit the penis. In retrograde ejaculation, the opening to the bladder does not close, allowing the semen to enter the bladder instead of exiting the penis. While this condition is not medically harmful, it does impair fertility [19].

Men with testicular cancer or colon cancer sometimes have surgery that can damage nerves involved in orgasm. The result may be a "dry orgasm," or the sensation of pleasure but without ejaculating any semen. Following a successful nerve-sparing radical prostatectomy, most men will have return of erections but will not be able to have children by natural means [20].

There should be no seminal fluid after the prostatectomy, so they will be "infertile" by natural means, but with in vitro fertilization techniques, it is still possible for a man to father a child after a radical prostatectomy. In this case intracytoplasmic sperm injection (ICSI) of single spermatozoon surgically recovered from the testis could lead to a pregnancy [21–23].

*Video: Sperm recovery after testicular sperm extraction (TESE)*https://www.youtube.com/watch?v=45W5XkzHy7w

Testicular cancer is associated with impaired spermatogenic function, even before orchiectomy, with a degree of dysfunction higher than that caused by local tumor effect [7].

Oligospermia is observed in more than 60 % of patients at the time of diagnosis of testicular cancer [8].

Storing sperm in a sperm bank before the operation is a recommended procedure for those men hoping to father children after the operation [24].

Last but not least, the vas deferens or the testicular blood supply may be injured or ligated at the time of inguinal surgery, hernia repair, hydrocelectomy, or varicocelectomy [25–27].

References

1. Meirow DA, Schenker JG (1995) Infertility: cancer and male infertility. Hum Reprod 10(8):2017–2022
2. Nudell DM, Monoski MM, Lipshultz LI (2002) Common medications and drugs: how they affect male fertility. Urol Clin North Am 29(4):965–973
3. Kuku SF, Oseghe DN (1989) Oligo/azoospermia in Nigeria. Arch Androl 22:233–238
4. Trasler JM, Hales BF, Robaire B (1986) Chronic low dose cyclophosphamide treatment of adult male rats: effect on fertility, pregnancy outcome and progeny. Biol Reprod 34(2): 275–283
5. DeVita VT, Hellman S, Rosenberg SA (2005) Cancer: principles & practice of oncology, 7th edn. Lippincott Williams & Wilkins, Philadelphia
6. Giwercman A, Petersen PM (2000) Cancer and male infertility. Baillieres Best Pract Res Clin Endocrinol Metab 14(3):453–471
7. Eisenberg ML, Betts P, Herder D, Lamb DJ, Lipshultz LI (2013) Increased risk of cancer among azoospermic men. Fertil Steril 100:681–685 [Medline]
8. Mulcahy N (2013) Male infertility increases overall cancer risk. Medscape Medical News. 21 June 2013. Available at http://www.medscape.com/viewarticle/806619. Accessed 30 July 2013
9. Carrol PR, Whitmore WF, Herr HW et al (1987) Endocrine and exocrine profiles of men with testicular tumors before orchiectomy. J Urol 137:420
10. Richie JP (1990) Clinical stage I testicular cancer: the role of modified retroperitoneal lymphadenectomy. J Urol 144:160
11. Lee SJ, Schover LR, Partridge AH et al (2006) American Society of Clinical Oncology recommendations on fertility preservation in cancer patients. J Clin Oncol 24:2917–2931
12. Raman JD, Nobert CF, Goldstein M (2005) Increased incidence of testicular cancer in men presenting with infertility and abnormal semen analysis. J Urol 174(5):1819–1822; discussion 1822
13. Beretta G, Zanollo A (1989) Intranasal gonadorelin in the treatment of cryptorchidism. Arch Ital Urol Nefrol Androl 61(3):333–335
14. Bouloux P, Warne DW, Loumaye E, FSH Study Group in Men's Infertility (2002) Efficacy and safety of recombinant human follicle-stimulating hormone in men with isolated hypogonadotropic hypogonadism. Fertil Steril 77(2):270–273
15. Beretta G, Fino E, Sibilio L, Dilena M (2005) Menotropin (hMG) and idiopathic oligoastenoteratozoospermia (OAT): effects on seminal fluid parameters and on results in ICSI cycles. Arch Ital Urol Androl 77(1):18–21
16. MacLeod J, Hotchkiss RS, Sitterson BW (1964) Recovery of male fertility after sterilization by nuclear radiation. JAMA 187(9):637–641
17. Houlgatte A, De La Taille A, Fournier R, Goluboff ET, Camporo P, Houdelette P (1999) Paternity in a patient with seminoma and carcinoma in situ in a solitary testis treated by partial orchidectomy. BJU Int 84(3):374–375
18. Jacobsen KD, Theodorsen L, Fossa SD (2001) Spermatogenesis after unilateral orchiectomy for testicular cancer in patients following surveillance policy. J Urol 165(1):93–96
19. Reynolds JC, McCall A, Kim ED, Lipshultz LI (1998) Bladder neck collagen injection restores antegrade ejaculation after bladder neck surgery. J Urol 159(4):1303
20. Jacobsen KD, Ous S, Waehre H, Trasti H, Stenwig AE, Lien HH et al (1999) Ejaculation in testicular cancer patients after post-chemotherapy retroperitoneal lymph node dissection. Br J Cancer 80(1–2):249–255
21. Palermo G, Joris H, Devroey P, Van Steirteghem AC (1992) Pregnancies after intracytoplasmic injection of single spermatozoon into an oocyte. Lancet 340(8810):17–18
22. Omurtag K, Cooper A, Bullock A et al (2013) Sperm recovery and IVF after testicular sperm extraction (TESE): effect of male diagnosis and use of off-site surgical centers on sperm recovery and IVF. PLoS One 8(7):e69838

23. Hauser R, Yogev L, Paz G, Yavetz H, Azem F, Lessing JB et al (2006) Comparison of efficacy of two techniques for testicular sperm retrieval in nonobstructive azoospermia: multifocal testicular sperm extraction versus multifocal testicular sperm aspiration. J Androl 27(1):28–33
24. Lewis R (2013) Freezing sperm a viable option in azoospermic men. Medscape Medical News [serial online]. 12 Aug 2013. Available at: http://www.medscape.com/viewarticle/809355. Accessed 28 Aug 2013
25. Zahalsky MP, Berman AJ, Nagler HM (2004) Evaluating the risk of epididymal injury during hydrocelectomy and spermatocelectomy. J Urol 171(6 Pt 1):2291–2292
26. Wantz GE (1984) Complications of inguinal hernia repair. Surg Clin North Am 64:287–1984
27. Beretta G (2005) Surgical treatment methods for obstructive azoospermia and surgical retrieve of spermatozoa for ICSI. Ital J Sex Reprod Med 3:159–165

Dietary Complements and Phytotherapy

16

Bruno Giammusso

Infertility is a major health problem affecting 15 % of couples in the reproductive age group. The male partner is contributory in up to 50 % cases and the cause of male infertility remains unknown in 25 % of men [1]. These men with idiopathic infertility are usually treated with a number of empirical therapies. The basis of the treatment is the fact that these products appear rational because of their mode of action or because of uncontrolled human studies [2]. Many over-the-counter (OTC) therapies have been historically used for male fertility, including herbs, vitamins, and nutritional supplements [3]. Many studies demonstrate the positive effects of OTC supplementation on semen parameters and pregnancy outcomes. Conversely, many studies also demonstrate a lack of improvement and potential complications with supplementation. Current and historical OTC medication studies suffer from a variety of drawbacks, including small short-duration studies, failure to perform randomized double-blinded placebo-controlled studies, and lack of standardization of dose and efficacy [4]. Definitive conclusions as to their true effects on male subfertility and dosing regimen could not be identified.

16.1 Antioxidants

Oxidative stress has been a well-studied aetiology of abnormal semen parameters [5–7]. Because of this, many of the current OTC therapies rely on antioxidant properties. Seminal oxidative stress (OS) results from an imbalance between reactive oxygen species (ROS) production and ROS scavenging by seminal antioxidants. Seminal OS is believed to be one of the main factors in the pathogenesis of sperm

B. Giammusso
Unità di Andrologia, Policlinico Morgagni, Via Vivante, 3, Catania 95123, Italy
e-mail: bgiammusso@hotmail.it

dysfunction and sperm DNA damage in male infertility [8–11]. It is estimated that 25 % of infertile men possess high levels of seminal ROS, whereas fertile men do not have high levels of seminal ROS [12, 13]. Spermatozoa are particularly susceptible to oxidative injury due to the abundance of plasma membrane polyunsaturated fatty acids [14–16]. Seminal oxidative stress has been related to infection, industrial exposure, tobacco use, and elevated temperature [7]. The two main sources for antioxidants are physiologic and dietary. Physiologic antioxidants are present within seminal plasma and the spermatozoa themselves [5]. If the high seminal ROS levels are due to a decreased ROS scavenging capacity of semen, it would support the use of dietary antioxidant supplementation [17]. A higher intake of antioxidants can potentially improve semen quality as well as sperm DNA integrity [18]. In contrast, poor semen quality may be associated with a lower intake and resultant lower concentration of antioxidants within the body [19]. The practice of prescribing oral antioxidant is supported by the lack of serious side effects related to antioxidant therapy, although few studies have carefully evaluated the risk of overtreatment with antioxidants [20]. Despite a large body of literature, it is not possible to establish firm conclusions regarding the optimal antioxidant treatment for infertile men because the published studies report on different types and doses of antioxidants, the studies are small, the end points vary, and few of the studies are placebo controlled [8, 13]. The most commonly studied oral antioxidants (or antioxidant enzyme cofactors) include vitamin E, vitamin C, carnitines, lycopene, glutathione, selenium, omega-3 and omega-6 fatty acids, zinc, arginine, and coenzyme-Q10.

16.2 Vitamin E

Vitamin E is a fat-soluble vitamin within the tocopherol family. It is a major lipophilic chain-breaking antioxidant known to inhibit free-radical–induced damage to cell membranes, protect tissue polyunsaturated fatty acids against peroxidation, and improve the activity of other antioxidants [21, 22]. Its antioxidant activity is similar to that of glutathione peroxidase. Therond et al. found that vitamin E is present in widely varying concentrations in human spermatozoa and semen plasma with the percent of motile spermatozoa significantly related to sperm α-tocopherol content [23]. Infertile men may have lower vitamin E in serum and seminal plasma [24]. Vitamin E is also effective in decreasing seminal ROS in infertile males [25, 26]. Substantial literature supports improvements in sperm motility, seminal ROS, and DNA fragmentation rates with vitamin E supplementation. Six RCTs evaluated the effects of vitamin E alone or in combination with vitamin C or selenium. Two of these studies reported a significant improvement in sperm motility [27, 28] and one reported a significant improvement in sperm DNA integrity [29] in the treatment arm only. In a randomized study of 54 infertile men, 28 were supplemented daily with 400 mg of vitamin E and 225 mcg selenium for 3 months, while the remaining 26 received 4–5 gm vitamin B daily for the same duration [28]. In contrast, three RCTs reported no significant improvement in sperm parameters after vitamin $E \pm C$ treatment [25, 30, 31]. Rolf et al. performed a placebo-controlled, double-blind study of high-dose oral vitamins C and E for 56 days in 31 infertile men with asthenozoospermia and a normal or only moderatedly decreased sperm concentration. Of the patients 15 received 1,000 mg vitamin C and 800 mg vitamin E, while 16 received placebo capsules. No changes occurred in semen parameters and no pregnancies were initiated.

16.3 Vitamin C

Vitamin C is a water-soluble vitamin that is an important cofactor for hydroxylation and amidation reactions. Vitamin C also functions as an important antioxidant and assists in recycling oxidized vitamin E [7]. It is highly concentrated within seminal plasma [32]. Vitamin C has been associated with various improvements in semen quality, although most studies have involved concurrent use of other vitamins and antioxidants. One RCT evaluated the effects of vitamin C alone and reported a significant improvement in sperm parameters in the treatment arm only [33]. Daily vitamin C supplementation with doses greater than 200 mg (up to 1,000 mg) was found to improve ($P<.05$) sperm count, motility, and viability in heavy smokers. A direct correlation was found between serum and seminal vitamin C concentrations and improvements in sperm quality, with those receiving 1,000 mg daily having the most improvements. These included improvements ($P<.05$) in count and viability of 34 %, motility of 5 %, and morphology of 33 % compared with baseline. Vitamin C plays an important role in protecting sperm and sperm DNA against oxidative damage by neutralizing ROS in a concentration-dependent manner [29]. Adequate vitamin C intake has also been shown to increase seminal vitamin C concentrations and reduce sperm DNA fragmentation [19, 34]. Greco demonstrated a reduction in DNA damage by 13 ($P<.001$) after treatment, as measured by terminal deoxyribonucleotidyl transferase–mediated dUTP nick-end labelling (TUNEL) assay [29]. Vitamin C is available in many fruits and vegetables [35]. The RDA is 90 mg to maintain body stores [36]. Side effects, occurring above the daily upper limit of 2,000 mg, include dyspepsia, headache, and increased risk of nephrolithiasis [35].

16.4 Carnitines

Carnitines are quaternary amines synthesized from the amino acids lysine and methionine. They are responsible for transporting long-chain fatty acids into the mitochondria for intracellular metabolism through β-oxidation. Carnitines assist sperm metabolism as an energy source for spermatozoa and affect motility and sperm maturation [37]. They have been proposed to have a role in sperm maturation during transit through the epididymis. They are also antioxidants protecting against ROS [38]. The two main forms of importance are L-carnitine (LC) and L-acetylcarnitine (LAC). Both are concentrated in the epididymis, spermatozoa, and seminal plasma [39]. Multiple randomized controlled studies supplementing with carnitine therapy for idiopathic infertility demonstrate improvements in concentration, motility, and morphology. Four RCTs evaluated the effects of L-carnitine alone or in combination with L-acetylcarnitine and three of the four reported a significant improvement in sperm parameters in the treatment arm only [40–43]. Lenzi et al. demonstrated significant improvements of total motile sperm count in the carnitine treatment arm, with an increase of 19 million ($P=.042$). The treatment group had a 13 % pregnancy rate compared with no pregnancies in the placebo group ($P>.05$) [44]. Balercia also demonstrated significant improvements with a 20–41 % increase in motility and a 13 % increase in morphology with LC or LAC supplementation or both for 24 weeks compared with placebo ($P<.05$) [40]. Nine pregnancies occurred in the treatment arms and three in the placebo arm ($P>.05$). Cavallini studied the effects of a combination of carnitine and cinnoxicam (nonsteroidal anti-inflammatory drug [NSAID]) therapy on sperm function [41]. Patients with no varicocele or small- or moderate-grade varicoceles treated with carnitine, alone or in combination with NSAID therapy, had significant improvements, with sperm concentration increases of 6–25 million/mL, motility increases of 2–22 %, and morphology increases of 8–23 % compared with placebo groups (P value not reported). Conversely, carnitine therapy has also been found to have nonsignificant effects on semen parameters by some investigators. Sigman et al. [43] performed a small randomized, double-blinded, placebo-controlled study on 21 patients. Patients were treated with carnitine therapy (2 g of LC and 1 g of LAC) or placebo daily for 24 weeks. At the end of the treatment period, there appeared to be a nonsignificant trend toward improvement in motility, with a 5.3 % increase in the treatment group compared with a 9.3 % increase in the placebo group ($P>.05$).

16.5 Lycopene

Lycopene is a powerful non-provitamin A carotenoid antioxidant that quenches singlet oxygen and scavenges peroxyl radicals. Its multiple roles include protection of lipid peroxidation, gap junction communication, cell growth regulation, gene expression modulation, and immune responses [45]. Palan and Naz measured seminal lycopene by high-pressure liquid chromatography in 37 men and noted significantly lower lycopene in the seminal plasma of immuno-infertile men than in fertile men [46]. Increased dietary intake or supplementation has been demonstrated to have positive effects on semen parameters [19]. Gupta and Kumar treated 30 infertile men with 4 mg lycopene for 3 months and found a significant improvement in sperm counts and motility with no significant changes in morphology. A 20 % pregnancy rate was seen during the course of the study [47].

16.6 Glutathione

Glutathione is the most abundant nonprotein thiol in mammalian cells. Glutathione reductases are selenoproteins. Glutathione is an endogenous antioxidant produced in the liver and is one of the most abundant antioxidants found in the body. It is a molecule synthesized from cysteine, glutamic acid, and glycine that plays an important role in maintaining exogenous antioxidants (i.e., vitamins C and E) in their active (reduced) roles [48]. The selenoprotein phospholipid hydroperoxide glutathione peroxidase occurs in the active form in spermatids. It reduces phospholipid hydroperoxide and scavenges hydrogen peroxide in human spermatozoa. Decreased phospholipid hydroperoxide glutathione peroxidase expression has been found in the spermatozoa of infertile men. Raijmakers et al. evaluated 25 men and found that fertile men had significantly higher glutathione in seminal fluid than subfertile men [49]. Significant associations of glutathione with sperm motility and sperm morphology were also observed. Ochsendorf et al. found that glutathione in the spermatozoa of patients with oligozoospermia was significantly lower than in controls [50]. Lenzi et al. [51, 52] have demonstrated improved sperm motility in infertile men with glutathione supplementation in multiple studies. They also treated men with varicoceles with intramuscular glutathione, noting a 10 % increase over baseline in total sperm motility with therapy ($P < .01$) [53]. Glutathione supplementation has been associated with improved sperm concentration and decreased sperm DNA fragmentation in a nonrandomized study using a combination of glutathione, vitamin C, and vitamin E [54]. Dietary sources of glutathione include fresh meat products, fruits, and vegetables [55].

16.7 Selenium

In human beings, the nutritional functions of selenium are achieved by 25 selenoproteins that have selenocysteine at their active centre [56]. In men, selenoprotein GPx4 is found in the mitochondria that make up the midpiece sheath of the sperm tail. In the early phase of spermatogenesis, GPx4, as a peroxidase, protects spermatozoa by its antioxidant function, whereas in the later phase, it forms cross-links with midpiece proteins to become a structural component of the mitochondrial sheath surrounding the flagellum, which is essential for sperm motility [57]. The selenium intake required for optimal activity and concentration of GPx4 and selenoprotein P is around 75 mcg per day. Supplementation might not be necessary if adequate daily intake is obtained through a diverse diet [58]. Selenium has been associated with positive effects on male infertility, which appear synergistic when used with other OTC supplements. Optimal dosing appears to be between 100 and 210 µg on the basis of the studies. In a randomized trial, selenium supplementation (100 mcg per day) of subfertile men with low selenium intake significantly increased sperm motility and enabled 11 % of the men to achieve paternity, compared with none in the placebo group [56]. However, high selenium intake (about 300 mcg per day) was shown to decrease sperm motility [59]. Selenium in combination with other antioxidants has been noted to improve sperm count, motility, and morphology [60]. Selenium deficiency has been found to decrease sperm motility, affect spermatozoa midpiece stability, and result in abnormal sperm morphology [61]. Multiple studies have demonstrated selenium's synergistic effects with other OTC supplements on sperm motility. In one prospective randomized study, infertile men with OAT receiving a 3-month course of selenium (210 µg) and vitamin E (400 mg) had a significant increase in sperm motility of 8 % ($P<.05$) and a decrease in lipid peroxidation levels, measured by an 8 % decrease in the malondialdehyde (MDA) level ($P<.05$) [28]. Three RCTs evaluated the effects of selenium alone or in combination with *N*-acetyl cysteine and two of the three studies reported a significant improvement in sperm parameters in the treatment arm only [60, 62, 63]. Contrary to the previous studies, one noncontrolled study treating 33 men with idiopathic infertility with 200 µg of selenium daily for 12 weeks noted no improvements in concentration, morphology, and motility despite increases in serum and seminal selenium levels [64].

16.8 Omega-3 and Omega-6 Fatty Acids

The significant effects of dietary fatty acids (FAs) on male fertility have been well documented both in animal and human studies [65, 66]. Polyunsaturated fatty acids (PUFAs) are essential FAs, because they cannot be synthesized by the human body. Docosahexaenoic acid (DHA), eicosapentaenoic acid (EPA), and α-linolenic acid are the main omega-3 PUFAs. Linoleic acid, γ-linolenic acid, and arachidonic acid (AA) are the main omega-6 PUFAs. The first mechanism by which omega-3 and omega-6 PUFAs affect spermatogenesis is by the incorporation into the spermatozoa cell membrane [67]. Omega-3 and omega-6 PUFAs are structural components of cell membranes [68]. The lipid bilayer of cellular membranes is maintained by the presence of these PUFAs [69]. The successful fertilization of spermatozoa depends on the lipids of the spermatozoa membrane [70]. Increased omega-6/omega-3 ratio in spermatozoa has also been implicated in impaired semen quality in oligozoospermic and/or asthenozoospermic men [71]. Safarinejad et al. [72] investigated PUFA composition of the blood plasma and spermatozoa in men with idiopathic OAT. They found that fertile men had higher blood and spermatozoa levels of omega-3 PUFAs compared with the infertile counterparts. Attaman et al. [73] evaluated the relation between dietary fats and semen quality in 99 men. They concluded that higher intake of omega-3 PUFAs was positively correlated with sperm morphology.

16.9 Zinc

Zinc has roles in testicular steroidogenesis, testicular development, spermatozoa oxygen consumption, nuclear chromatin condensation, the acrosome reaction, acrosin activity, sperm chromatin stabilization, and conversion of testosterone to 5α-dihydrotestosterone [74]. The male genitourinary tract has a high concentration of zinc, especially in the prostate. Chronic mild zinc deficiency is associated with oligospermia, decreased serum testosterone levels, and compromised immune system function [75]. Five RCTs evaluated the effects of zinc alone or in combination with folic acid and all five reported a significant improvement in sperm parameters in the treatment arm only [60, 76–81]. Young studied the association of folate, zinc, and antioxidant intake with sperm aneuploidy in 89 healthy nonsmoking men through a dietary and supplement questionnaire and sperm FISH studies [18]. In a controlled study 45 infertile men with asthenozoospermia were treated with three different regimens of zinc—200 mg orally twice daily with or without vitamin C, vitamin E for 3 months, and both regimens—compared with controls [78]. Zinc therapy with or without additional vitamins was associated with increases in sperm motility of at least 24 % ($P<.001$).

16.10 Arginine

Arginine is a biologic precursor of nitric oxide. In the male reproductive system, arginine is a biochemical precursor for synthesizing spermidine and spermine and is thought to be essential for sperm motility [82]. Multiple studies have evaluated arginine's effect on semen. Some studies have reported that supplementation up to 4 g/day improves sperm concentration and motility [83, 84], whereas others have failed to demonstrate improvement in semen parameters or pregnancy rates [85, 86].

16.11 Coenzyme Q-10

Coenzyme Q-10 (CoQ10) plays a key role in transporting electrons in the mitochondrial respiratory chain [87]. It stabilizes and protects the cell membrane from oxidative stress [88]. CoQ10 levels are measurable within seminal fluid and can be directly correlated with sperm count and motility [89]. In a placebo-controlled, double-blinded, randomized controlled study, Balercia et al. [90] treated men with idiopathic subfertility with decreased motility (<50 %) with CoQ10. There was a 6 % absolute motility improvement in the treatment group after 6 months of treatment compared with the placebo group ($P<.0001$) although no difference in pregnancy rates. In a placebo-controlled study, Safarinejad [91] demonstrated absolute increases in total sperm count of 9.8 %, motility of 4.5 %, and morphology of 1.8 % over baseline with CoQ10 therapy when compared with placebo ($P=.01$).

16.12 Phytotherapy

Herbal therapy is increasingly popular worldwide as a way to treat infertility. In the United States, 17 % constantly visited herbal therapies in the past 18 months out of the 29 % of infertile couples who use complementary and alternative medicine [92]. Ginseng is one of the most popular herbs used in the phytotherapy of male infertility. Both oligoasthenospermic patients and age-matched healthy counterpart showed an increase in spermatozoa density and motility after the use of *Panax ginseng* [93]. Asthenospermic patients treated with ginseng also showed a significant increase in progressive sperm motility [94]. In the last few years Maca, a perennial plant of the *Lepidium meyenii* species, has been extensively studied for its pharmacological properties on human spermatogenesis. An open-label study conducted by administering daily 1,500–3,000 mg of Maca for 4 months resulted in increased seminal volume, sperm count, and sperm motility [95]. A strong natural lipophilic antioxidant, astaxanthin, has been studied in a prospective, double-blind, randomized trial, designed to evaluate the effect of 16 mg/day astaxanthin compared to placebo in 30 infertile men. At the end of the study, ROS and inhibin B decreased significantly and sperm linear velocity increased in the treated group. The total and per cycle pregnancy rates among the placebo cases (10.5 and 3.6 %) were lower compared with 54.5 and 23.1 %, respectively, in the astaxanthin group ($P=0.028$; $P=0.036$) [96].

References

1. Siddiq FM, Sigman M (2002) A new look at the medical management of infertility. Urol Clin North Am 29:949–963
2. Kumar R, Gautam G, Gupta NP (2006) Drug therapy for idiopathic male infertility: rationale versus evidence. J Urol 176:1307–1312
3. Ko EY, Sabanegh ES (2012) The role of over-the-counter supplements for the treatment of male infertility – fact or fiction? J Androl 33:292–308
4. Agarwal A, Sekhon LH (2010) The role of antioxidant therapy in the treatment of male infertility. Hum Fertil 13:217–225
5. Tremellen K (2008) Oxidative stress and male infertility—a clinical perspective. Hum Reprod Update 14:243–258
6. Agarwal A, Sharma RK, Desai NR et al (2009) Role of oxidative stress in pathogenesis of varicocele and infertility. Urology 73:461–469
7. Kefer JC, Agarwal A, Sabanegh E (2009) Role of antioxidants in the treatment of male infertility. Int J Urol 16:449–457
8. Zini A, San Gabriel M, Baazeem A (2009) Antioxidants and sperm DNA damage: a clinical perspective. J Assist Reprod Genet 26:427–432
9. Aitken RJ, de Iuliis GN, Finnie JM et al (2010) Analysis of the relationships between oxidative stress, DNA damage and sperm vitality in a patient population: development of diagnostic criteria. Hum Reprod 25:2415–2426
10. Fraga CG, Motchnik PA, Shigenaga MK et al (1991) Ascorbic acid protects against endogenous oxidative DNA damage in human sperm. Proc Natl Acad Sci U S A 88:11003–11006
11. Iwasaki A, Gagnon C (1992) Formation of reactive oxygen species in spermatozoa of infertile patients. Fertil Steril 57:409–416
12. Zini A, Sigman M (2009) Are tests of sperm DNA damage clinically useful? Pros and cons. J Androl 30:219–229
13. Agarwal A, Nallella KP, Allamaneni SS et al (2004) Role of antioxidants in treatment of male infertility: an overview of the literature. Reprod Biomed Online 8:616–627
14. Aitken RJ, Clarkson JS (1987) Cellular basis of defective sperm function and its association with the genesis of reactive oxygen species by human spermatozoa. J Reprod Fertil 81:459–469
15. de Lamirande E, Gagnon C (1992) Reactive oxygen species and human spermatozoa. I. Effects on the motility of intact spermatozoa and on sperm axonemes. J Androl 13:368–378
16. Zini A, Garrels K, Phang D (2000) Antioxidant activity in the semen of fertile and infertile men. Urology 55:922–926
17. Lewis SE, Boyle PM, McKinney KA et al (1995) Total antioxidant capacity of seminal plasma is different in fertile and infertile men. Fertil Steril 64:868–870
18. Young SS, Eskenazi B, Marchetti FM et al (2008) The association of folate, zinc, and antioxidant intake with sperm aneuploidy in healthy non-smoking men. Hum Reprod 23:1014–1022

19. Mendiola J, Torres-Cantero AM, Vioque J et al (2010) A low intake of antioxidant nutrients is associated with poor semen quality in patients attending fertility clinics. Fertil Steril 93:1128–1133
20. Henkel RR (2011) Leukocytes and oxidative stress: dilemma for sperm function and male fertility. Asian J Androl 13:43–52
21. Palamanda JR, Kehrer JR (1993) Involvement of vitamin E and protein thiols in the inhibition of microsomal lipid peroxidation by glutathione. Lipids 23:427–443
22. Brigelius-Flohé R, Traber MG (1999) Vitamin E: function and metabolism. FASEB J 13:1145–1155
23. Therond P, Auger J, Legrand A et al (1996) Alpha-tocopherol in human spermatozoa and seminal plasma: relationships with motility, antioxidant enzymes and leucocytes. Mol Hum Reprod 2:739–741
24. Omu AE, Fatinikun T, Mannazhath N et al (1999) Significance of simultaneous determination of serum and seminal plasma α–tocopherol and retinol in infertile men by high-performance liquid chromatography. Andrologia 31:347–351
25. Kessopoulou E, Powers HJ, Sharma KK et al (1995) A double-blind randomized placebo crossover controlled trial using the antioxidant vitamin E to treat reactive oxygen species associated male infertility. Fertil Steril 64:825–831
26. Ross C, Morriss A, Khairy M et al (2010) A systematic review of the effect of oral antioxidants on male infertility. Reprod Biomed Online 20:711–723
27. Suleiman SA, Ali ME, Zaki ZM et al (1996) Lipid peroxidation and human sperm motility: protective role of vitamin E. J Androl 17:530–537
28. Keskes-Ammar L, Feki-Chakroun N, Rebai T et al (2003) Sperm oxidative stress and the effect of an oral vitamin E and selenium supplement on semen quality in infertile men. Arch Androl 49:83–94
29. Greco E, Iacobelli M, Rienzi L et al (2005) Reduction of the incidence of sperm DNA fragmentation by oral antioxidant treatment. J Androl 26:349–353
30. Moilanen J, Hovatta O, Lindroth L (1993) Vitamin E levels in seminal plasma can be elevated by oral administration of vitamin E in infertile men. Int J Androl 16:165–166
31. Rolf C, Cooper TG, Yeung CH et al (1999) Antioxidant treatment of patients with asthenozoospermia or moderate oligoasthenozoospermia with high-dose vitamin C and vitamin E: a randomized, placebo-controlled, double-blind study. Hum Reprod 14:1028–1033
32. Dawson EB, Harris WA, Rankin WE et al (1987) Effect of ascorbic acid on male fertility. Ann N Y Acad Sci 498:312–323
33. Dawson EB, Harris WA, Teter MC et al (1992) Effect of ascorbic acid supplementation on the sperm quality of smokers. Fertil Steril 58:1034–1039
34. Colagar AH, Marzony ET (2009) Ascorbic acid in human seminal plasma: determination and its relationship to sperm quality. J Clin Biochem Nutr 45:144–149
35. Alpers DH, Stenson WF, Taylor BE, Bier DM (eds) (2008) Manual of nutritional therapeutics, 5th edn. Lippincott Williams & Wilkins, Philadelphia
36. Standing Committee on the Scientific Evaluation of Dietary Reference Intakes, Food and Nutrition Board, Institute of Medicine (2000) Dietary reference intakes for vitamin C, vitamin E, selenium, and beta-carotene and other carotenoids. National Academies Press, Washington, DC
37. Palmero S, Bottazzi C, Costa M et al (2000) Metabolic effects of l-carnitine on prepubertal rat Sertoli cells. Horm Metab Res 32:87–90
38. Vicari E, La Vignera S, Calogero A (2002) Antioxidant treatment with carnitines is effective in infertile patients with prostatovesiculoepididymitis and elevated seminal leukocyte concentrations after treatment with nonsteroidal anti-inflammatory compounds. Fertil Steril 6:1203–1208
39. Bohmer T, Hoel P, Purvis K et al (1978) Carnitine levels in human accessory sex organs. Arch Androl 1:53–59
40. Balercia G, Regoli F, Armeni T et al (2005) Placebo-controlled double-blind randomized trial on the use of L-carnitine, L-acetylcarnitine, or combined L-carnitine and L-acetylcarnitine in men with idiopathic asthenozoospermia. Fertil Steril 84:662–671

41. Cavallini G, Ferraretti AP, Gianaroli L et al (2004) Cinnoxicam and L-carnitine/acetyl–carnitine treatment for idiopathic and varicocele-associated oligoasthenospermia. J Androl 25:761–770; discussion 71–72
42. Lenzi A, Lombardo F, Sgro P et al (2003) Use of carnitine therapy in selected cases of male factor infertility: a double-blind crossover trial. Fertil Steril 79:292–300
43. Sigman M, Glass S, Campagnone J et al (2006) Carnitine for the treatment of idiopathic asthenospermia: a randomized, double-blind, placebo-controlled trial. Fertil Steril 85:1409–1414
44. Lenzi A, Sgro P, Salacone P et al (2004) A placebo-controlled double-blind randomized trial in the use of combined l-carnitine and l-acetylcarnitine treatment in men with asthenozoospermia. Fertil Steril 81:1578–1584
45. Rao AV, Mira MR, Rao LG (2006) Lycopene. Adv Food Nutr Res 51:99–164
46. Palan P, Naz R (1996) Changes in various antioxidant levels in human seminal plasma related to immunoinfertility. Arch Androl 36:139–148
47. Gupta NP, Kumar R (2002) Lycopene therapy in idiopathic male infertility—a preliminary report. Int Urol Nephrol 34:369–372
48. Irvine DS (1996) Glutathione as a treatment for male infertility. Rev Reprod 1:6–12
49. Raijmakers MT, Roelofs HM, Steegers EA et al (2003) Glutathione and glutathione S-transferases A1-1 and P-P1 in seminal plasma may play a role in protecting against oxidative damage to spermatozoa. Fertil Steril 79:169–175
50. Ochsendorf FR, Buhl R, Bastlein A et al (1998) Glutathione in spermatozoa and seminal plasma of infertile men. Hum Reprod 13:353–357
51. Lenzi A, Lombardo F, Gandini L et al (1992) Glutathione therapy for male infertility. Arch Androl 29:65–68
52. Lenzi A, Picardo M, Gandini L et al (1994) Glutathione treatment of dyspermia: effect on the lipoperoxidation process. Hum Reprod 9:2044–2050
53. Lenzi A, Culasso F, Gandini L et al (1993) Placebo-controlled, double blind, cross-over trial of glutathione therapy in male infertility. Hum Reprod 8:1657–1662
54. Kodama H, Yamaguchi R, Fukuda J et al (1997) Increased oxidative deoxyribonucleic acid damage in the spermatozoa of infertile male patients. Fertil Steril 68:519–524
55. Jones DP, Coates RJ, Flagg EW et al (1992) Glutathione in foods listed in the National Cancer Institute's Health Habits and History Food Frequency Questionnaire. Nutr Cancer 17:57–75
56. Rayman MP (2000) The importance of selenium to human health. Lancet 356:233–241
57. Ursini F, Heim S, Kiess M et al (1999) Dual function of the selenoprotein PHGPx during sperm maturation. Science 285:1393–1396
58. Xia Y, Hill KE, Li P et al (2010) Optimization of selenoprotein P and other plasma selenium biomarkers for the assessment of the selenium nutritional requirement: a placebo-controlled, double-blind study of selenomethionine supplementation in selenium-deficient Chinese subjects. Am J Clin Nutr 92:525–531
59. Hawkes WC, Turek PJ (2001) Effects of dietary selenium on sperm motility in healthy men. J Androl 22:764–772
60. Safarinejad MR, Safarinejad S (2009) Efficacy of selenium and/or N-acetylcysteine for improving semen parameters in infertile men: a double-blind, placebo controlled, randomized study. J Urol 181:741–751
61. Watanabe T, Endo A (1991) Effects of selenium deficiency on sperm morphology and spermatocyte chromosomes in mice. Mutat Res 262:93–99
62. Scott R, MacPherson A, Yates RW et al (1998) The effect of oral selenium supplementation on human sperm motility. Br J Urol 82:76–80
63. Hawkes WC, Alkan Z, Wong K (2009) Selenium supplementation does not affect testicular selenium status or semen quality in North American men. J Androl 30:525–533
64. Iwanier K, Zachara BA (1995) Selenium supplementation enhances the element concentration in blood and seminal fluid but does not change the spermatozoal quality characteristics in subfertile men. J Androl 16:441–447
65. Bongalhardo DC, Leeson S, Buhr MM (2009) Dietary lipids differentially affect membranes from different areas of rooster sperm. Poult Sci 88:1060–1069

66. Tavilani H, Doosti M, Abdi K et al (2006) Decreased polyunsaturated and increased saturated fatty acid concentration in spermatozoa from asthenozoospermic males as compared with normozoospermic males. Andrologia 38:173–178
67. Safarinejad MR, Safarinejad S (2012) The roles of omega-3 and omega-6 fatty acids in idiopathic male infertility. Asian J Androl 14:514–515
68. Mazza M, Pomponi M, Janiri L et al (2007) Omega-3 fatty acids and antioxidants in neurological and psychiatric diseases: an overview. Prog Neuropsychopharmacol Biol Psychiatry 31:12–26
69. Farooqui AA, Horrocks LA, Farooqui T (2000) Glycerophospholipids in brain: their metabolism, incorporation into membranes, functions, and involvement in neurological disorders. Chem Phys Lipids 106:1–29
70. Lenzi A, Gandini L, Maresca V et al (2000) Fatty acid composition of spermatozoa and immature germ cells. Mol Hum Reprod 6:226–231
71. Aksoy Y, Aksoy H, Altinkaynak K et al (2006) Sperm fatty acid composition in subfertile men. Prostaglandins Leukot Essent Fatty Acids 75:75–79
72. Safarinejad MR, Hosseini SY, Dadkhah F et al (2010) Relationship of omega-3 and omega-6 fatty acids with semen characteristics, and anti-oxidant status of seminal plasma: a comparison between fertile and infertile men. Clin Nutr 29:100–105
73. Attaman JA, Toth TL, Furtado J et al (2012) Dietary fat and semen quality among men attending a fertility clinic. Hum Reprod 27:1466–1474
74. Ebisch IM, Thomas CM, Peters WH et al (2007) The importance of folate, zinc and antioxidants in the pathogenesis and prevention of subfertility. Hum Reprod 13:163–174
75. Prasad AS (2008) Zinc in human health: effect of zinc on immune cells. Mol Med 14:353–357
76. Ebisch IM, Pierik FH, de Jong FH et al (2006) Does folic acid and zinc sulphate intervention affect endocrine parameters and sperm characteristics in men. Int J Androl 29:339–345
77. Mahajan SK, Abbasi AA, Prasad AS et al (1982) Effect of oral zinc therapy on gonadal function in hemodialysis patients. A double-blind study. Ann Intern Med 97:357–361
78. Omu AE, Al-Azemi MK, Kehinde EO et al (2008) Indications of the mechanisms involved in improved sperm parameters by zinc therapy. Med Princ Pract 17:108–116
79. Omu AE, Dashti H, Al-Othman S (1998) Treatment of asthenozoospermia with zinc sulphate: andrological, immunological and obstetric outcome. Eur J Obstet Gynecol Reprod Biol 79:179–184
80. Piomboni P, Gambera L, Serafini F et al (2008) Sperm quality improvement after natural antioxidant treatment of asthenoteratospermic men with leukocytospermia. Asian J Androl 10:201–206
81. Wong WY, Merkus HM, Thomas CM et al (2002) Effects of folic acid and zinc sulfate on male factor subfertility: a double-blind, randomized, placebo-controlled trial. Fertil Steril 77:491–498
82. Sinclair S (2000) Male infertility: nutritional and environmental considerations. Altern Med Rev 5:28–38
83. Schachter A, Goldman JA, Zukerman Z (1973) Treatment of oligospermia with the amino acid arginine. J Urol 110:311–313
84. de Aloysio D, Mantuano R, Mauloni M et al (1982) The clinical use of arginine aspartate in male infertility. Acta Eur Fertil 13:133–167
85. Miroueh A (1970) Effect of arginine on oligospermia. Fertil Steril 21:217–219
86. Pryor JP, Blandy JP, Evans P et al (1978) Controlled clinical trial of arginine for infertile men with oligozoospermia. Br J Urol 50:47–50
87. Hidaka T, Fujii K, Funahashi I et al (2008) Safety assessment of coenzyme Q10 (CoQ10). Biofactors 32:199–208
88. Bentinger M, Tekle M, Dallner G (2010) Coenzyme Q—biosynthesis and functions. Biochem Biophys Res Commun 396:74–79
89. Mancini A, de Marinis L, Oradei A et al (1994) Coenzyme Q10 concentrations in normal and pathological human seminal fluid. J Androl 15:591–594

90. Balercia G, Buldreghini E, Vignini A et al (2009) Coenzyme Q10 treatment in infertile men with idiopathic asthenozoospermia: a placebo-controlled, double-blind randomized trial. Fertil Steril 91:1785–1792
91. Safarinejad MR (2009) Efficacy of coenzyme Q10 on semen parameters, sperm function and reproductive hormones in infertile men. J Urol 182:237–248
92. Smith JF, Eisenberg ML, Millstein SG et al (2010) The use of complementary and alternative fertility treatment in couples seeking fertility care: data from a prospective cohort in the United States. Fertil Steril 93:2169–2174
93. Salvati G, Genovesi G, Marcellini L et al (1996) Effects of Panax Ginseng C.A. Meyer saponins on male fertility. Panminerva Med 38:249–254
94. Morgante G, Scolaro V, Tosti C et al (2010) Treatment with carnitine, acetyl carnitine, L-arginine and ginseng improves sperm motility and sexual health in men with asthenospermia. Minerva Urol Nefrol 62:213–218
95. Gonzales GF, Cordova A, Gonzales C et al (2001) Lepidium meyenii (Maca) improved semen parameters in adult men. Asian J Androl 3:301–303
96. Comhaire FH, El Garem Y, Mahmoud A et al (2005) Combined conventional/antioxidant "Astaxanthin" treatment for male infertility: a double blind, randomized trial. Asian J Androl 7:257–262

Environmental Pollution and Infertility

17

Giorgio Cavallini

17.1 Introduction

A decline in sperm counts has emerged in recent years [1–3]. Consequently, it has been argued that male fertility is declining, and it is further proposed that environmental pollutants may play an active role [4–10]. By contrast, no apparent and clear decrease in population fertility has been noted in epidemiologic studies [11, 12]. Decline in sperm count of healthy men of reproductive age over the years has been higher in some regions (Denmark, Scotland, USA east coast) than in others (USA west coast, south of France, Baltic countries). Genetic and racial factors may also be involved [7–12].

It has been hypothesized that environmental chemicals with estrogenic properties, heavy metals, and solvents constitute detrimental factors for sperm count [13–18], even though the epidemiologic consequences are unclear. Nevertheless, some kind of toxicologic effect on spermatogenesis is hypothesized; clinical and laboratory research indicates that of all the changes in male reproductive health seem to be interrelated and may have a common origin in fetal life or childhood [19–23]. Furthermore, some epidemiologic studies confirm that exposure to endocrine disruptors, solvents, and heavy metals may play a role in male reproductive disorders [24].

Three categories of potential reproductive disruptor pollutants have been found: endocrine disruptors, heavy metals, and organic solvents.

G. Cavallini
Andrological Section, Gynepro-Medical Team,
via Tranquillo Cremona 8, 40137 Bologna, Italy
e-mail: giorgiocavallini@libero.it

17.2 Endocrine Disruptors

Endocrine disruptors affect the male genital tract during fetal testis and germinal cell development (testicular dysgenesis syndrome), targeting pituitary gonadotropins [25] or the genetic regulation of steroidogenesis [26] at either the genomic [27] or proteomic [28, 29] levels. Gene pathways targeted include cholesterol transport and steroidogenesis, pathways involved in intracellular cholesterol/lipid homeostasis, insulin signaling, transcriptional regulation, oxidative stress [27], α-inhibin (which is essential for physiologic Sertoli cell development), and genes involved with communication between Sertoli cells and gonocytes [27]. Environmental pollutants are thought to induce oxidative stress, peroxidation [30], and germ cell apoptosis in the human fetal testis [31].

There exists a critical period of exposure: diethylstilbestrol (an estrogenic compound) exposure during the perinatal period can influence behavior, accessory glands, and reproductive structures in humans and rodents [32] via hormonal or epigenetic mechanisms [33].

Given that animals represent an accepted experimental model for human male reproduction, it is noteworthy that pollutants are regarded as etiologic factors in the reproductive decline of wildlife [34, 35]. Perinatal exposure is critical for the development of testicular dysgenesis syndrome in animals [36–38]. A severe problem of pollutants is that some of these chemicals have long half-lives and have been detected in environmental samples 10–20 years after they were banned for use [39].

Pesticides, fungicides, heavy metals, defoliants, and other chemical weapons, in addition to oils and cleaning agents [40–44], are regarded as the main environmental pollutants capable of disrupting the human and wildlife endocrine system (endocrine disruptor chemicals or EDCs).

Endocrine disruption is a mechanism of toxicity that hinders the ability of cells, tissues, and organs to communicate hormonally [45], provoking reduced fertility and fecundity [17], spontaneous abortion, skewed sex ratios [46], male and female reproductive tract abnormalities [47–49], precocious puberty [50, 51], polycystic ovary syndrome [52], neurobehavioral disorders, impaired immune function, and a wide variety of cancers [53, 54]. Endocrine disruptors represent a wide range of chemical classes and include agonists of the estrogen receptor, androgen receptor antagonists, and aryl hydrocarbon receptor agonists [55]. Some chemicals have more than one mechanism of action [56]. A list of endocrine disruptors is shown in Table 17.1. Many of these chemicals persist in the environment. Some are lipophilic and, hence, sequestered in adipose tissue and secreted in milk, whereas others may only be present for short periods of time but at critical periods of development.

17.3 Heavy Metals

All heavy metals are toxic and can affect the seminiferous epithelium [57–59]. Cadmium interacts with the zinc-dependent stability of the human sperm chromatin [60]. Salts of arsenic, cadmium, mercury, lead, and antimony are all toxic for

Table 17.1 Environmental pollutants: their sources and health effects [66]

Pollutant	Origin	Health effects During development	Health effects During adulthood
[a]Bisfenol A	Component of polycarbonate plastic and epoxy resins	Modified prostate development and puberty onset, hormonal changes, decreased semen quality, obesity	Decreased semen and oocyte quality, recurrent miscarriages
[a]Dioxin/furans	Manufacture or burning of products containing chlorine	Urologic malformations	Menstrual irregularities, epigenetic disorders
[a]Organochlorine pesticides	Largely banned in Western countries, still persist in the food chain (DDT)	Altered sex ratio, altered puberty onset, decreased semen quality	Altered puberty onset, decreased semen quality, endometriosis, fetal loss
[a]Pentachlorophenol	Wood preservative, railroad ties	Reduced fertility	Reduced fertility
[a]Ethylene oxide	Chemical sterilizer for dental practice	?	Decreased semen quality, miscarriage
[a]Glycol ethers	Paints, enamels, wood stains; printing inks, cosmetics	?	Reduced fertility, decreased semen quality, fetal loss, menstrual irregularities
[a]Nonylphenol, octylphenol	Detergents, pesticides, paints, plasticizers	Hormonal changes, altered puberty onset, decreased testicular size, decreased semen quality	?
[a]Perfluorinated compounds	Water-repellent treatments	Hormonal changes, fetal loss, reduced birth weight	?
[a]Phthalates	Cosmetics, toys, lubricants	Malformations of reproductive tract, hormonal changes, decreased semen quality	Earlier menarche, menstrual irregularities, endometriosis, ovulation alterations, decreased semen quality, fetal loss
[a]Polybrominated diphenyl esters	Flame retardants	?	Decreased semen quality
[b]Mercury	Thermometers, dental filling	Decreased semen quality	Decreased semen quality
[b]Cadmium	Batteries, pigments, some metal alloys	Sertoli cell and testicle damage	Toxic to Sertoli cells and spermatogenesis
[b]Lead	Batteries, ammunition, metal products, X-ray shields	Hormonal and pubertal onset alterations	Hormonal alterations, menstrual alterations, reduced fertility, fetal loss, altered puberty, reduced spermatogenesis

(continued)

Table 17.1 (continued)

Pollutant	Origin	Health effects	
		During development	During adulthood
[b]Manganese	Dietary supplements, ceramics, pesticides, fertilizers	Hormonal changes, altered puberty onset	Hormonal changes, menstrual irregularities, fetal loss, altered puberty onset, damage to Sertoli cells and spermatogenesis
Organic solvents: benzene, toluene, 1-bromopropane, 2-bromopropane, perchloroethylene, trichloroethylene, etc	Plastic, resin, rubbers, synthetic fibers, lubricants, dyes, detergents, drugs, pesticides, fingernail polish, cleaning products, detergents, lacquers, fiberglass, food containers	Hormonal changes, pubertal onset alterations, reduced fertility, menstrual irregularities, miscarriage and fetal loss, decreased semen quality	Hormonal changes, reduced fertility, menstrual irregularities, miscarriage and fetal loss, decreased semen quality

[a]Chlorinated hydrocarbons (endocrine disruptors)
[b]Heavy metals

spermatogenesis in humans and animal models [61, 62]. Heavy metals are also present in some welding fluxes [63].

17.4 Solvents

Various organic solvents are also known to cause infertility, including glycol ethers [64], which are used in the printing industry and are also found in some paints (e.g., as used on naval vessels). Perchloroethylene, used in the dry cleaning industry, can also cause subfertility, but its effects on sperm morphology and kinematics are subtle, and their impact on fertility remains unclear [65].

References

1. Carlsen E, Giwercman A, Keiding N, Skakkebaek NE (1992) Evidence for decreasing quality of semen during past 50 years. BMJ 305:609–613
2. Sharpe RM, Skakkebaek NE (1993) Are oestrogens involved in falling sperm count and disorders of the male reproductive tract? Lancet 341:1392–1395
3. Sharpe RM (2012) Sperm counts and fertility in men: a rocky road ahead. Science & Society Series on Sex and Science. EMBO Rep 13:398–403
4. Perry MJ (2008) Effects of environmental and occupational pesticide exposure on human sperm: a systematic review. Hum Reprod Update 14:233–242
5. Jurewicz J, Hanke W, Radwan M, Bonde JP (2009) Environmental factors and semen quality. Int J Occup Med Environ Health 22:305–329
6. European Science Foundation (2010) Male reproductive health. Its impacts in relation to general wellbeing and low European fertility rates. Science Policy Briefing 40 http://www.esf.org/publications/science-policy-briefings.html

7. Joffe M (2010) What has happened to human fertility? Hum Reprod 25:295–307
8. Sharpe RM (2010) Environmental/lifestyle effects on spermatogenesis. Philos Trans R Soc Lond B Biol Sci 365:1697–1712
9. Perry MJ, Venners SA, Chen X, Liu X, Tang G, Xing H, Barr DB, Xu X (2011) Organophosphorous pesticide exposures and sperm quality. Reprod Toxicol 31:75–79
10. Sutton P, Woodruff TJ, Perron J, Stotland N, Conry JA, Miller MD, Giudice LC (2012) Toxic environmental chemicals: the role of reproductive health professionals in preventing harmful exposures. Am J Obstet Gynecol 207:164–173
11. Akre O, Cnattingius S, Bergström R, Kvist U, Trichopoulos D, Ekbom A (1999) Human fertility does not decline: evidence from Sweden. Fertil Steril 71:1066–1069
12. Scheike TH, Rylander L, Carstensen L, Keiding N, Jensen TK, Stromberg U, Joffe M, Akre O (2008) Time trends in human fecundability in Sweden. Epidemiology 19:191–196
13. Tas S, Lauwerys R, Lison D (1996) Occupational hazards for the male reproductive system. Crit Rev Toxicol 26:261–307
14. Van Waeleghem K, De Clercq N, Vermeulen L, Schoonjans F, Comhaire F (1996) Deterioration of sperm quality in young healthy Belgian men. Hum Reprod 11:325–329
15. Phillips KP, Tanphaichitr N (2008) Human exposure to endocrine disrupters and semen quality. J Toxicol Environ Health B Crit Rev 11:188–220
16. Diamanti-Kandarakis E, Bourguignon JP, Giudice LC, Hauser R, Prins GS, Soto AM, Zoeller RT, Gore AC (2009) Endocrine-disrupting chemicals: an Endocrine Society scientific statement. Endocr Rev 30:293–342
17. Giwercman A (2011) Estrogens and phytoestrogens in male infertility. Curr Opin Urol 21:519–526
18. Woodruff TJ (2011) Bridging epidemiology and model organisms to increase understanding of endocrine disrupting chemicals and human health effects. J Steroid Biochem Mol Biol 127:108–117
19. Sharpe RM (2006) Pathways of endocrine disruption during male sexual differentiation and masculinisation. Best Pract Res Clin Endocrinol Metab 20:91–110
20. Sharpe RM, Skakkebaek NE (2003) Male reproductive disorders and the role of endocrine disruption: advances in understanding and identification of areas for future research. Pure Appl Chem 75:2023–2038
21. Skakkebaek NE, Toppari J, Söder O, Gordon M, Divall S, Draznin M (2011) The exposure of fetuses and children to endocrine disrupting chemicals: a European Society for Paediatric Endocrinology (ESPE) and Pediatric Endocrine Society (PES) call to action statement. J Clin Endocrinol Metab 96:3056–3058
22. Skakkebaek NE, Rajpert-De-Meyts E, Main KM (2001) Testicular dysgenesis syndrome: an increasingly common developmental disorder with environmental aspects. Hum Reprod 16:972–978
23. Buck Louis GM, Gray LE Jr, Marcus M, Ojeda SR, Pescovitz OH, Witchel SF, Sippell W, Abbott DH, Soto A, Tyl RW (2008) Environmental factors and puberty timing: expert panel research needs. Pediatrics 112:192–207
24. Scott HM, Mason JI, Sharpe RM (2009) Steroidogenesis in the fetal testis and its susceptibility to disruption by exogenous compounds. Endocr Rev 30:883–925
25. Mutoh J, Taketoh J, Okamura K, Kagawa T, Ishida T, Ishii Y, Yamada H (2006) Fetal pituitary gonadotropin as an initial target of dioxin in its impairment of cholesterol transportation and steroidogenesis in rats. Endocrinology 147:927–936
26. Kuhl AJ, Ross SM, Gaido KW (2007) CCAAT/enhancer binding protein beta, but not steroidogenic factor-1, modulates the phthalate-induced dysregulation of rat fetal testicular steroidogenesis. Endocrinology 148:5851–5864
27. Liu K, Lehmann KP, Sar M, Young SS, Gaido KW (2005) Gene expression profiling following in utero exposure to phthalate esters reveals new gene targets in the etiology of testicular dysgenesis. Biol Reprod 73:180–192
28. Laier P, Metzdorff SB, Borch J, Hagen ML, Hass U, Christiansen S, Axelstad M, Kledal T, Dalgaard M, McKinnell C (2006) Mechanisms of action underlying the antiandrogenic effects of the fungicide prochloraz. Toxicol Appl Pharmacol 213:160–171

29. Klinefelter GR, Laskey JW, Winnik WM, Suarez JD, Roberts NL, Strader LF, Riffle BW, Veeramachaneni DN (2012) Novel molecular targets associated with testicular dysgenesis induced by gestational exposure to diethylhexyl phthalate in the rat: a role for estradiol. Reproduction 144:747–761
30. Kabuto H, Amakawa M, Shishibori T (2004) Exposure to bisphenol A during embryonic/fetal life and infancy increases oxidative injury and causes underdevelopment of the brain and testis in mice. Life Sci 74:2931–2940
31. Coutts SM, Fulton N, Anderson RA (2007) Environmental toxicant-induced germ cell apoptosis in the human fetal testis. Hum Reprod 22:2912–2918
32. Harris RM, Waring RH (2012) Diethylstilboestrol—a long-term legacy. Maturitas 72:108–112
33. Anway MD, Memon MA, Uzumcu M, Skinner MK (2006) Transgenerational effect of the endocrine disruptor vinclozolin on male spermatogenesis. J Androl 27:868–879
34. Edwards TM, Moore BC, Guillette LJ Jr (2006) Reproductive dysgenesis in wildlife: a comparative view. Int J Androl 29:109–121
35. Hamlin HJ, Guillette LJ (2010) Birth defects in wildlife: the role of environmental contaminants as inducers of reproductive and developmental dysfunction. Syst Biol Reprod Med 56:113–121
36. Danish Environmental Protection Agency (1995) Male reproductive health and environmental chemicals with estrogenic effects. Ministry of Environment and Energy, Danish Environmental Protection Agency, Copenhagen; Miljoproject 290
37. Toppari J, Larsen J, Christiansen P, Giwercman A, Grandjean P, Guillette LJ Jr, Jégou B, Jensen TK, Jouannet P, Keiding N (1996) Male reproductive health and environmental xenoestrogens. Environ Health Perspect 104(Suppl 4):741–803
38. Braw-Tal R (2010) Endocrine disruptors and timing of human exposure. Pediatr Endocrinol Rev 8:41–46
39. Aitken RJ, Koopman P, Lewis SEM (2004) Seeds of concern. Nature 432:48–52
40. Colborn T, vom Saal FS, Soto AM (1993) Developmental effects of endocrine-disrupting chemicals in wildlife and humans. Environ Health Perspect 101:378–384
41. Colborn T, Dumanoski D, Myers JP (1997) Our stolen future: are we threatening our fertility, intelligence, and survival?—A scientific detective story. Plume/Penguin Books USA, New York
42. Sheiner EK, Sheiner E, Hammel RD, Potashnik G, Carel R (2003) Effect of occupational exposures on male fertility: literature review. Ind Health 41:55–62
43. Gore AC (2007) Endocrine-disrupting chemicals: from basic research to clinical practice. Humana Press, Totowa
44. Woodruff TJ, Carlson A, Schwartz JM, Guidice LC (2008) Proceedings of the summit on environmental challenges to reproductive health and fertility: executive summary. Fertil Steril 89:281–300
45. Silva LF, Felipe V, Cavagna M, Pontes A, Baruffi RL, Oliveira JB (2012) Large nuclear vacuoles are indicative of abnormal chromatin packaging in human spermatozoa. Int J Androl 35:46–51
46. Yiee JH, Baskin LS (2010) Environmental factors in genitourinary development. J Urol 180:34–41
47. Bornman MS, Barnhoorn IEJ, de Jager C, Veeramachaneni DNR (2010) Testicular microlithiasis and neoplastic lesions in wild eland (*Tragelaphus oryx*): possible effects of exposure to environmental pollutants? Environ Res 110:327–333
48. Newbold RR (2011) Developmental exposure to endocrine-disrupting chemicals programs for reproductive tract alterations and obesity later in life. Am J Clin Nutr 94:1939S–1942S
49. Dunbar B, Patel M, Fahey J, Wira C (2012) Endocrine control of mucosal immunity in the female reproductive tract: impact of environmental disruptors. Mol Cell Endocrinol 354:85–93

50. Mouritsen A, Aksglaede L, Sørensen K, Mogensen SS, Leffers H, Main KM, Frederiksen H, Andersson AM, Skakkebaek NE, Juul A (2010) Hypothesis: exposure to endocrine-disrupting chemicals may interfere with timing of puberty. Int J Androl 33:346–359
51. Deng F, Tao FB, Li DY, Xu YY, Hao JH, Sun Y (2012) Effects of growth environments and two environmental endocrine disruptors on children with idiopathic precocious puberty. Eur J Endocrinol 166:803–809
52. Teede H, Deeks A, Moran L (2010) Polycystic ovary syndrome: a complex condition with psychological, reproductive and metabolic manifestations that impacts on health across the lifespan. BMC Med 8:41–51
53. Keinan-Boker L, van Der Schouw YT, Grobbee DE, Peeters PH (2004) Dietary phytoestrogens and breast cancer risk. Am J Clin Nutr 79:282–288
54. Ndebele K, Graham B, Tchounwou PB (2010) Estrogenic activity of coumestrol, DDT, and TCDD in human cervical cancer cells. Int J Environ Res Public Health 7:2045–2056
55. Beischlag TV, Luis MJ, Hollingshead BD, Perdew GH (2008) The aryl hydrocarbon receptor complex and the control of gene expression. Crit Rev Eukaryot Gene Expr 18:207–250
56. Phillips KP, Foster WG (2008) Key developments in endocrine disrupter research and human health. J Toxicol Environ Health B Crit Rev 11:322–344
57. Bonde JP (2010) Male reproductive organs are at risk from environmental hazards. Asian J Androl 12:152–156
58. Wirth JJ, Mijal RS (2010) Adverse effects of low level heavy metal exposure on male reproductive function. Syst Biol Reprod Med 56:147–167
59. Marzec-Wróblewska U, Kamiński P, Lakota P (2012) Influence of chemical elements on mammalian spermatozoa. Folia Biol 58:7–15
60. Casswall TH, Björndahl L, Kvist U (1987) Cadmium interacts with the zinc-dependent stability of the human sperm chromatin. J Trace Elem Electrolytes Health Dis 1:85–87
61. Boscolo P, Sacchattoni-Longrocino G, Ranelletti FO, Gioia A, Carmignani M (1985) Effects of long term cadmium exposure on the testes of rabbits: ultrastructural study. Toxicol Lett 24:145–149
62. Benoff S, Cooper GW, Hurley I, Mandel FS, Rosenfeld DL, Scholl GM, Gilbert BR, Hershlag A (1994) The effect of calcium ion channel blockers on sperm fertilization potential. Fertil Steril 62:606–617
63. Lynch E, Braithwaite R (2005) A review of the clinical and toxicological aspects of 'traditional' (herbal) medicines adulterated with heavy metals. Expert Opin Drug Saf 4:769–778
64. Cherry N, Moore H, McNamee R, Pacey A, Burgess G, Clyma JA, Dippnall M, Baillie H, Povey A (2008) Occupation and male infertility: glycol ethers and other exposures. Occup Environ Med 65:708–714
65. Eskenazi B, Wyrobek AJ, Fenster L, Katz DF, Sadler M, Lee J, Hudes M, Rempel DM (1991) A study of the effect of perchloroethylene exposure on semen quality in dry cleaning workers. Am J Ind Med 20:575–591
66. Mortimer D, Barratt CL, Björndahl L, de Jager C, Jequier AM, Muller CH (2013) What should it take to describe a substance or product as 'sperm-safe'. Hum Reprod Update 19(Suppl 1): 1–45

The Role of the Andrologist in Assisted Reproduction

18

Giorgio Cavallini and Giovanni Beretta

18.1 Background

Article 1 of 40/2004 of the Italian law [1] states that assisted reproduction techniques (ARTs) should be started only when any other therapy for infertility has failed. In some cases any attempt to improve spermatogenesis is useless; in others its improvement increases the probabilities of an ART take-home baby.

18.2 Specific Indications for ART

Any medical or surgical therapy for male infertility is useless in the following cases; thus, ART should be immediately started.

18.3 Globozoospermia

Globozoospermia, the so-called roundheaded syndrome, is a sperm defect of low frequency (incidence <0.1 % of infertile patients) but is associated with a severe teratozoospermia causing male sterility [2]. Globozoospermia is characterized by the absence of acrosome in roundheaded spermatozoa, leading to a complete inability

---

G. Cavallini (✉)
Andrological Section, Gynepro-Medical Group,
via Tranquillo Cremona 8, Bologna 40137, Italy
e-mail: giorgiocavallini@libero.it

G. Beretta
Andrological and Reproductive Medicine Unit, Centro Demetra,
via Della Fortezza 6, Firenze 50129, Italy
e-mail: giovanniberetta@libero.it

© Springer International Publishing Switzerland 2015
G. Cavallini, G. Beretta (eds.), *Clinical Management of Male Infertility*,
DOI 10.1007/978-3-319-08503-6_18

to fertilize the oocyte; thus the affected males suffer from infertility. A genetic basis was suggested by the familial distribution of the syndrome [3], and different modes of inheritance have been described [4, 5].

18.3.1 Female Ageing

The size of the initial oocyte stock, the proportion that undergoes atresia, and the rate of initiation of growth of follicles are genetically determined variables. The number of oocytes in the ovaries declines naturally and progressively through the process of atresia, and fecundity declines gradually beginning at the age of 32 and even more rapidly after 37 years [6].

Anti-Müllerian hormone (AMH) correlates with the number of antral follicles and has been recently identified as an early reliable predictor of ovarian reserve [7, 8]. This data means that improvement of sperm count is useless when female partner is >40 years [9] and that correction of mild dyspermias is ineffective for natural conception when female partner is >35 [10] or in any case in which AMH and AFC (antral follicle count) are strongly reduced independently of the female age. Anyway andrological clinic evaluation and scrotal ultrasounds are necessary to verify the presence or the absence of a testicular cancer.

18.3.2 Micropolycystic Ovary

Polycystic ovary syndrome is a heterogeneous endocrine disorder found in 5 % of women of reproductive age and accounts for about 90–95 % of patients with anovulatory infertility. This syndrome presents defects in primary cellular control mechanisms that result in the expression of chronic anovulation, hyperandrogenism, and polycystic ovaries. Some studies employing DNA microarrays have identified over one thousand genes whose expression was altered in PCOS patients. These provide evidence that the genetic abnormality in PCOS affects key mechanisms of follicular development and steroidogenesis, resulting in increased ovarian androgen secretion and anovulatory infertility due to arrested folliculogenesis. These data means that gametes of women affected by polycystic ovary syndrome are too severely compromised to have their ART performance increased with a spermatogenesis improvement [11].

18.3.3 Presence of Y Microdeletions and/or High Follicle-Stimulating Hormone (FSH) >12 mIU/ml)

Short arm Y chromosome microdeletion and high FSH are laboratory signs of a spermatogenesis that is too compromised to be improved by any medical or surgical approach [12–14].

18.3.4 Unexplained Male Infertility

See Chap. 10.

18.3.5 Congenital Absence of the Vas Deferens

See Chap. 5.

18.4 Specific Indications to Improve Spermatogenesis Before ART

An attempt to improve spermatogenesis should be performed in all other cases.

In fact complementary treatment with antioxidant-containing food supplements quadruples the spontaneous pregnancy rate and reduces the cost per pregnancy by 60 % [15]. Any andrological treatment lowers the number of couples who need ART for pregnancy [16].

In nonobstructive azoospermic (NOA) patients, the probabilities to conceive are directly linked to the monitors of spermatogenesis: sperm motility, testicular histology, follicle-stimulating hormone (FSH) level, previous testicular pathology, and number of sperm retrieved [17–20].

Gonadotropin supplementation of hypogonadal oligoasthenoteratospermic (OAT) patients improves sperm count and intracellular sperm injection (ICSI) offsprings [21, 22]. Patients who had their sperm count improved after a varicocele ligation seldom achieved a spontaneous pregnancy; however, they had greater probabilities of a take-home baby after ICSI than the patients who had no sperm ejaculated after varicocelectomy and who were submitted to (micro-)testicular sperm extraction [23]. The numbers of ICSI pregnancies and live births in severe idiopathic OAT patients improved with a course of L-carnitine, acetyl-L-carnitine, and cinnoxicam. The improvement occurred in the patients who had their sperm aneuploidy reduced and their sperm morphology increased [24]. Further varicocele correction presents a possible method to optimize a couples' reproductive potential increasing ICSI offspring or decreasing the need for complex assisted reproductive technology [25].

Approximately 5 % of children born through ICSI are at an increased risk of chromosomal anomalies because of the de novo aberrations (aneuploidies) that arise during gametogenesis of their parents. This percentage is much higher than the expected value of 0.5 % in the general population [26, 27]. Thus a correction of spermatogenesis might lower the percentages of chromosome anomalies of spermatozoa and of children born after ICSI.

Actually intracytoplasmic morphologically selected sperm injection (IMSI) [28] or injection of spermatozoa which have undergone to acrosome [29] reaction is a valuable option for patients with severe male factors to improve ICSI offsprings; however, a correct andrological approach to OAT decreases the need of complex reproductive technology [25, 30].

References

1. Parlamento della repubblica Italiana. Legge 19 febbraio 2004, n. 40, "Norme in materia di procreazione medicalmente assistita". Gazzetta Ufficiale n. 45 del 24 febbraio 2004
2. Schirren C, Holstein A, Schirren C (1971) Uber die Morphogenese rundkopfiger Spermatozoen des Menschen. Andrologie 3:117–125
3. Kilani ZM, Shaban MA, Ghunaim SD, Keilani SS, Dakkak AI (1998) Triplet pregnancy and delivery after intracytoplasmic injection of round-headed spermatozoa. Hum Reprod 13:2177–2179
4. Dam AH, Koscinski I, Kremer JA, Moutou C, Jaeger AS, Oudakker AR, Tournaye H, Charlet N, Lagier-Tourenne C, van Bokhoven H (2007) Homozygous mutation in SPATA16 is associated with male infertility in human globozoospermia. Am J Hum Genet 81:813–820
5. Dam AH, Ramos L, Dijkman HB, Woestenenk R, Robben H, van den Hoven L, Kremer JA (2011) Morphology of partial globozoospermia. J Androl 32:199–206
6. Alviggi C, Humaidan P, Howles CM, Tredway D, Hillier SG (2009) Biological versus chronological ovarian age: implications for assisted reproductive technology. Reprod Biol Endocrinol 7:101–108
7. Barad DH, Weghofer A, Gleicher N (2009) Comparing anti-Müllerian hormone (AMH) and follicle-stimulating hormone (FSH) as predictors of ovarian function. Fertil Steril 91:1553–1555
8. La Marca A, Sighinolfi G, Radi D, Argento C, Baraldi E, Artenisio AC (2010) Anti-müllerian hormone (AMH) as a predictive marker in assisted reproductive technology (ART). Hum Reprod Update 16:113–130
9. Sunderam S, Kissin DM, Flowers L, Anderson JE, Folger SG, Jamieson DJ, Barfield WD, Centers for Disease Control and Prevention (CDC) (2012) Assisted reproductive technology surveillance–United States, 2009. MMWR Surveill Summ 61:1–23
10. Schlegel PN (2012) Contemporary issues in varicocele management. Curr Opin Urol 22:487–488
11. de Resende LO, Vireque AA, Santana LF, Moreno DA, De Sá Rosa e Silva AC, Ferriani RA, Scrideli CA, Reis RM (2012) Single-cell expression analysis of BMP15 and GDF9 in mature oocytes and BMPR2 in cumulus cells of women with polycystic ovary syndrome undergoing controlled ovarian hyperstimulation. J Assist Reprod Genet 29:1057–1065
12. Choi DK, Gong IH, Hwang JH, Oh JJ, Hong JY (2013) Detection of Y chromosome microdeletion is valuable in the treatment of patients with nonobstructive azoospermia and oligoasthenoteratozoospermia: sperm retrieval rate and birth rate. Korean J Urol 54:111–116
13. Sagnak L, Ersoy H, Ozok U, Eraslan A, Yararbas K, Goktug G, Tukun A (2010) The significance of Y chromosome microdeletion analysis in subfertile men with clinical varicocele. Arch Med Sci 6:382–387
14. Matzuk MM, Lamb DJ (2008) The biology of infertility: research advances and clinical challenges. Nat Med 14:1197–1213
15. Comhaire F, Decleer W (2011) Quantifying the effectiveness and cost-efficiency of food supplementation with antioxidants for male infertility. Reprod Biomed Online 23:361–362
16. Comhaire F, Decleer W (2012) Comparing the effectiveness of infertility treatments by numbers needed to treat (NNT). Andrologia 44:401–404
17. Dafopoulos K, Griesinger G, Schultze-Mosgau A, Orief Y, Schopper B (2005) Factors affecting outcome after ICSI with spermatozoa retrieved from cryopreserved testicular tissue in non obstructive azoospermia. Reprod Biomed Online 10:455–460
18. de Croo I, van der Elst J, Everaert K, de Sutter P, Dhont M (2000) Fertilization, pregnancy and embryo implantation rates after ICSI in cases of obstructive and non-obstructive azoospermia. Hum Reprod 15:1383–1388
19. Zitzmann M, Nordhoff V, von Schonfeld V, Nordsiek-Mengede A, Kliesch S (2006) Elevated follicle stimulating hormone levels and the chances for azoospermic men to become fathers after retrieval of elongated spermatids from cryopreserved testicular tissue. Fertil Steril 86:339–347

20. Cavallini G, Cristina Magli M, Crippa A, Resta S, Vitali G, Pia Ferraretti A, Gianaroli L (2011) The number of spermatozoa collected with testicular sperm extraction is a novel predictor of intracytoplasmic sperm injection outcome in non-obstructive azoospermic patients. Asian J Androl 13:312–316
21. Anawalt BD (2013) Approach to male infertility and induction of spermatogenesis. J Clin Endocrinol Metab 98:3532–3542
22. Beretta G, Fino E, Sibilio L, Dilena M (2005) Menotropin (hMG) and idiopathic oligoastenoteratozoospermia (OAT): effects on seminal fluid parameters and on results in ICSI cycles. Arch Ital Urol Androl 77:18–21
23. Weedin JW, Khera M, Lipshultz LI (2010) Varicocele repair in patients with nonobstructive azoospermia: a meta-analysis. J Urol 183:2309–2315
24. Cavallini G, Magli MC, Crippa A, Ferraretti AP, Gianaroli L (2012) Reduction in sperm aneuploidy levels in severe oligoasthenoteratospermic patients after medical therapy: a preliminary report. Asian J Androl 14:591–598
25. McIntyre M, Hsieh TC, Lipshultz L (2012) Varicocele repair in the era of modern assisted reproductive techniques. Curr Opin Urol 22:517–520
26. Bonduelle M, Liebaers I, Deketelaere V, Derde VM, Camus M et al (2002) Neonatal data on a cohort of 2889 infants born after ICSI (1991–1999) and of 2995 infants born after IVF (1983–1999). Hum Reprod 17:671–694
27. Hindryckx A, Peeraer K, Debrock S, Legius E, de Zegher F (2010) Has the prevalence of congenital abnormalities after intracytoplasmic sperm injection increased? The Leuven data 1994–2000 and a review of the literature. Gynecol Obstet Invest 29:11–22
28. El Khattabi L, Dupont C, Sermondade N, Hugues JN, Poncelet C, Porcher R, Cedrin-Durnerin I, Lévy R, Sifer C (2013) Is intracytoplasmic morphologically selected sperm injection effective in patients with infertility related to teratozoospermia or repeated implantation failure? Fertil Steril 100:62–68
29. Gianaroli L, Magli MC, Ferraretti AP, Crippa A, Lappi M, Capitani S, Baccetti B (2010) Birefringence characteristics in sperm heads allow for the selection of reacted spermatozoa for intracytoplasmic sperm injection. Fertil Steril 93:807–813
30. Cavallini G, Ferraretti AP, Gianaroli L, Biagiotti G, Vitali G (2004) Cinnoxicam and L-carnitine/acetyl-L-carnitine treatment for idiopathic and varicocele-associated oligoasthenospermia. J Androl 25:761–770

Sexual Problems and Infertility

19

Giovanni Beretta

19.1 Epidemiology

It is estimated that male factor infertility is the main or a contributing cause of infertility in half of involuntarily childless couples [1].

Infertility is an emotional crisis and a physical challenge because it interferes with one of the most fundamental human activities. From a list of 87 items of stressful life events, infertility has been ranked as one of the most stressful situations similar to the death of a spouse or of a close relative [2].

This stressful condition frequently causes diminished sexual desire as a side effect of feelings of sexual unattractiveness, guilt, shame, depression and anger or can be the consequence of the stress and demands infertility places on the marriage, social relationships, work life and financial resources. Infertility frequently triggers feelings of failure, sexual inadequacy, diminished masculinity and altered sense of self, and all are contributory factors in male sexual dysfunction. Many men develop performance anxiety; sexual avoidance especially if sex is for "procreation purpose only" and the female partners have become sexually irresponsive and passive.

Sexual dysfunction is more openly discussed than in the past, but still only a fraction of the men with these problems seek medical care [3].

After sexual desire disorder the most common sexual problem is erectile failure in 5–10 % of the general male population, 4–10 % inhibited male orgasm in 35 % premature ejaculation [4].

The relationship between sexual dysfunctions and infertility can be mutual. Sexual dysfunction may cause difficulty conceiving but also attempts to conceive may cause sexual dysfunctions.

G. Beretta
Andrological and Reproductive Medicine Unit, Centro Demetra,
via Della Fortezza 6, 50129 Firenze, Italy
e-mail: giovanniberetta@libero.it

19.2 Sexual Dysfunction Causing Infertility

For a small percentage of infertile couples, male sexual problems are the main cause of infertility [5]. For others it could be a relative cause: If a couple cannot or does not have sex near ovulation time, the woman is less likely to get pregnant. If they have sex once in a while because of low sexual desire or pain during sex, they may miss that important time for pregnancy.

19.3 Erectile Dysfunction

It is traditionally referred to as impotence, and the NIH consensus conference has defined erectile dysfunction (ED) as the inability to achieve or maintain an erection adequate for sexual intercourse. Primary erectile failure is never having had the ability to achieve and/or maintain an erection sufficient for vaginal penetration or successful coitus. This condition is very rare but, when it does occur, is a direct cause of infertility. Treatment success rates for primary erectile dysfunction are the lowest among all sexual disorders in men and women.

Secondary erectile dysfunction is partial or weak erections, total absence of an erection or the inability to sustain erections long enough for vaginal penetration or sexual intercourse. Most men experience some form of episodic, transient erectile dysfunction at some point of their lifetime, especially when they age, although it affects men of all ages [6]. Years ago it was believed that the main cause of erectile dysfunctions was due to psychological factors, but nowadays it is believed that at least 50 % of erectile dysfunction problems are due to organic aetiology [7].

The pathophysiology of erectile dysfunction may be vascular, neurogenic, hormonal, anatomical, drug induced or psychogenic [6].

Erectile dysfunction is the most important cause of male factor infertility due to sexual dysfunction, although men rarely disclose this problem to caregivers [8]. In one study, 10 % of men were observed to experience sexual dysfunction of a psychogenic nature in response to the diagnosis of infertility [9].

The introduction of new oral therapies has completely changed the diagnostic and therapeutic approach to ED, and the current availability of effective and safe drugs for ED has resulted in an increasing number of men seeking help for ED. These patients may benefit from a prescription of a PDE-5 inhibitor. Neither sildenafil nor tadalafil has an adverse effect on sperm function or ejaculate quality [10, 11].

Patients who complain of difficulty with ejaculation and climax may be taking psychotherapeutic agents that block dopamine production and consequently blunt the hypothalamic-pituitary axis and possibly decrease libido. Other psychotherapeutic drugs can decrease vasodilation and worsen the quality of erections.

When ED is determined to be organic and not reversible (in case of injury or disease), treatment could involve intracavernous injection or surgical interventions such as penile prostheses [12]. Psychological treatments include decreasing performance anxiety, increasing awareness of erotic sensations and disputing irrational belief and myths.

19.4 Premature Ejaculation

Premature ejaculation (PE) is an extremely common condition. Kinsey, in his landmark report, had stated that it affects as many as 70 % of all men. PE is characterized by a lack of voluntary control over ejaculation. Many men occasionally ejaculate sooner than they or their partner would like during sexual activities. PE is a frustrating problem that can reduce the enjoyment of sex, harm relationships and affect quality of life. When it comes to conception, there are two things that must happen – intercourse with vaginal penetration and ejaculation. When the latter happens first, it will impact fertility, but only in those rare cases in which ejaculation happens before the introduction of the penis in the vagina. PE is usually not situational; it occurs with all partners because the men have not learned to voluntary control his ejaculatory reflexes [13]. Although the exact cause of premature ejaculation (PE) is not known, new studies suggest that serotonin, a natural substance produced by nerves, is important [14].

A breakdown of the actions of serotonin in the brain may be a cause. Studies have found that high amounts of serotonin in the brain slow the time to ejaculation, while low amounts of serotonin can produce a condition like PE.

Psychological factors also commonly contribute to PE. Temporary depression, stress, unrealistic expectations about performance, a history of sexual repression or an overall lack of confidence can cause PE. Interpersonal dynamics may contribute to sexual function. PE can be caused by a lack of communication between partners, hurt feelings or unresolved conflicts that interfere with the ability to achieve emotional intimacy. These psychological factors may be related to infertility with its emphasis on sex for procreation.

There are several treatment choices for premature ejaculation: psychological therapy, behavioural therapy and medications [15].

19.5 Inhibited or Delayed Ejaculation

Inhibited or delayed ejaculation (also called retarded ejaculation) is the persistent and recurrent inhibition of orgasm, manifested by delay or absence of ejaculation following adequate sexual stimulation; the most frequent physical situation which interferes with ejaculation is spinal cord injury; researchers report that ejaculation occurs in up to 70 % of men with incomplete lower-level injuries and in as many as 17 % of men with complete lower-level injuries. Ejaculation occurs in about 30 % of men with incomplete upper-level injuries and almost never in men with complete upper-level injuries [16].

These conditions prevent men from ejaculating during sexual intercourse even though they can often ejaculate normally through masturbation. The causes could be psychological and physical; psychological anejaculation is usually anorgasmic and it could be situational or total. Situational means that men can ejaculate in some conditions or situation but not in others. It also can occur in stressful situations, as when a man is asked to collect a sperm sample in an infertility laboratory. Recently, delayed ejaculation has been identified as a common side effect of some antidepressant medications [17].

Treatments depend on the cause and include psychosexual counselling and drugs as ephedrine and imipramine. When delayed ejaculation affects fertility, vibrator or electroejaculation (a procedure in which ejaculation is stimulated by low electrical current) or surgical retrieval of sperm directly from the testis can be used to obtain sperm for insemination or used in IVF [18].

19.6 Infertility as a Cause of Sexual Dysfunction

Infertility can negatively influence both the pleasure of sex and sexual function. In many couples, sexuality has already been compromised before infertility treatment because of the failure to conceive and the subsequent medical interventions [19]. The invasion of the couple's physical and emotional privacy during fertility treatments can further reduce sexual desire in both partners and damage the relationship [20].

Men are sensitive of the stress of infertility techniques as intrauterine insemination (IUI) and in vitro fertilization (IVF); this can be due to a diminished sense of male self-esteem. It has also been shown that the emotional stress of the men enrolled in the IVF programmes can negatively affect the quality of semen [21]. Moreover, the "super stress" of the moment, "this is the night" syndrome and the necessity to perform can deteriorate sexual performance and cause erectile failure. Some procedures such as the post-coital test are particularly involved in the impairment of sexual functioning [22].

When infertility results in relationship disturbances and sexual problems, the intervention of a caregiver is paramount. All too often the sexual problems of infertile couples are ignored and minimized in a belief that they will dissipate on their own or will have a few long-term consequences. Unfortunately these beliefs are not true: although some sexual problems may disappear when the pressures of infertility treatment end, sexual difficulties typically linger or become more problematic after treatment ends or parenthood is achieved [23]. Professional attention and care regarding sexual disturbances during infertility can lower the impact, and education can prevent many of the sexual difficulties infertile couples encounter. The European Society of Human Reproduction and Embryology (ESHRE) has set up specific guidelines in order to provide a framework for counselling in infertility being aware that sexual counselling is dependent upon the legal, ethical and cultural background of every country [24].

References

1. McLachlan RI, de Kretser DM (2001) Male infertility: the case for continued research. Med J Aust 174:116–117
2. Dohrenwend BS, Dohrenwend BP (1981) Stressful life events (their nature and effect). Wiley, New York

3. Zanollo A, Beretta G, Zanollo L (1991) Anamnestic criteria for sexual evaluation in the andrological field. Arch Ital Urol Nefrol Androl 63(4):493–497
4. Simons JS, Carey MP (2001) Prevalence of sexual dysfunctions: results from a decade of research. Arch Sex Behav 30:177–219
5. Mimoun S (1993) The multiple interactions between infertility and sexuality. Contracept Fertil Sex 21(3):251–254
6. Lewis RW (2001) Epidemiology of erectile dysfunction. Urol Clin North Am 28:209–216
7. Bain J (1993) Sexuality and infertility in the male. Can J Hum Sex 2:157–160
8. Andrews FM, Abbey A, Halman J (1991) Stress from infertility, marriage factors and subjective well-being of wives and husbands. J Health Soc Behav 32:238–253
9. Saleh RA, Ranga GM, Raina R (2003) Sexual dysfunction in men undergoing infertility evaluation: a cohort observational study. Fertil Steril 79:909–912
10. Purvis K, Muirhead GJ, Harness JA (2002) The effects of Sildenafil on human sperm function in healthy volunteers. Br J Clin Pharmacol 53(Suppl 1):53S–60S
11. Hellstrom WJ, Overstreet JW, Yu A (2003) Tadalafil has no detrimental effect on human spermatogenesis or reproductive hormones. J Urol 170:887–889
12. Beretta G, Zanollo A, Portaluppi W (1991) Intracavernous injections of prostaglandin E1 in the treatment of erection disorders. Arch Ital Urol Nefrol Androl 63(4):481–485
13. Kaplan HS (1983) Evaluation of sexual disorders: psychological and medical aspects. Brunner/Mazel, New York
14. Giuliano F, Clement P (2006) Serotonin and premature ejaculation: from physiology to patient management. Eur Urol 50:454–466
15. Beretta G, Chelo E, Fanciullacci F, Zanollo A (1986) Effect of an alpha-blocking agent (phenoxybenzamine) in the management of premature ejaculation. Acta Eur Fertil 17(1):43–45
16. Zanollo A, Marzotto M, Politi P, Spinelli M, Beretta G (1995) Management of sexual dysfunction in spinal cord injury. Arch Ital Urol Androl 67(5):315–319
17. Waldinger MD, Quinn P, Dilleen M, Mundayat R, Schweitzer DH, Boolell M (2005) Original research-ejaculation disorders: a multinational population survey of intravaginal ejaculation latency time. J Sex Med 22:492–497
18. Hendry WF (1998) Disorders of ejaculation: congenital, acquired and functional. Br J Urol 82:331–341
19. Coeffin-Driol C, Giami A (2004) L'impact de l'infertilité et de ses traitements la vie sexuelle et la relation de couple: revue de la literature. Gynecol Obstet Fertil 32:624–637
20. Leiblum SR, Aviv A, Hammer R (1998) Life after infertility treatment: a long term investigation of marital and sexual function. Hum Reprod 13:3569–3574
21. Ragni G, Caccamo A (1992) Negative effect of stress of in vitro fertilization program on quality of semen. Acta Eur Fertil 23:21–23
22. Boivin J, Takefman JE, Brender W, Tulandi T (1992) The effects of sexual response in coitus on early reproductive processes. J Behav Med 15(5):509–551
23. Burns LH (1995) An overview of sexual dysfunction in the infertile couple. J Fam Psychother 6:25–46
24. Boivin J, Appleton TC, Baetens P, Baron J, Bitzer J et al (2001) Guidelines for counselling in infertility: outline version. Hum Reprod 16(6):1301–1304

Index

A
Adamopoulos, D.A., 110
Agbaje, I.M., 92
Al-Kandari, A.M., 58
Antiestrogen, 95, 140
Antioxidant, 59, 82, 84, 93–95, 112, 153–157, 159, 160, 175
Arginine, 154, 159
Aromatase inhibitors, 85, 95, 141
Assisted reproduction, 1, 23, 30, 31, 34, 85, 173–175
Astaxanthin, 160
Asthenozoospermia, 7, 16, 155, 159
Attaman, J.A., 92, 158
Azoospermia, 15, 16, 26–28, 31, 41–52, 65, 67–69, 106, 111, 136, 137, 141, 146–149

B
Balercia, G., 156, 159
Beretta, G., 1–2, 13–19, 55–60, 145–149, 173–175, 179–182

C
Cavallini, G., 1–2, 33–37, 79–85, 99–102, 105–112, 156, 165–168, 173–175
Chavarro, J.E., 92
Chromosomal abnormalities, 63, 64, 67, 99, 101
Coenzyme Q-10 (CoQ10), 159
Colombo, F., 119–132
Comhaire, A., 56
Cryptorchidism, 7, 9, 23, 27, 44–46, 68, 69, 71, 83, 119–132, 136

D
DeCastro, B.J., 125
Diagnosis, 8, 13, 23–31, 35, 46–47, 57–58, 64–72, 82–83, 94–95, 99, 100, 102, 107–112, 120, 123, 124, 126, 128, 131, 139–140, 146, 149, 180

E
Eisenberg, M.L., 7, 92
El-Bayoumi, M.A., 112
Endocrine disruptors, 135, 138, 165, 166, 168
Enviromental pollution, 81, 94, 165–168
Erectile dysfunctions, 9, 93, 180
Etiology, 8, 33, 56–57, 63–64, 79–80, 84, 99–102, 107, 125, 153, 180
Evers, J.H., 59

F
Fariello, R.M., 92
Female age, 30, 34, 174
Franceschelli, A., 119–132
Franco, G., 41–52

G
Genetic screening, 47, 101
Genome, 18, 29, 68, 80, 101
Gentile, G., 119–132
Giammusso, B., 153–160
Ginseng, 159
Globozoospermia, 173–175
Glutathione, 154, 156–157
Gupta, N.P., 156

H

Harrison, R.M., 56
Hauser, R., 51
Heavy metals, 82, 94, 165–168
Herbal therapy, 159
Hofny, E.R., 92
Hu, Y.Y., 112

I

Idiopathic infertility, 8, 69, 153, 156, 158
Idiopathic oligoasthenoteratospermia, 83
Inhibited or delayed ejaculation., 181–182
Intracytoplasmic morphologically selected sperm injection (IMSI), 175
Intracytoplasmic sperm injection (ICSI), 44, 48–51, 66, 149, 175

J

Jensen, T.K., 92
Jungwirth, A., 8

K

Kinsey, 19
Klinefelter, H.F., 8, 27, 44, 63–66, 68, 125, 136
Kruger, T.F., 16
Kumar, R., 156

L

Laboratory procedures, 5, 14, 26, 50, 79, 95, 102, 165, 174, 182
L-acetylcarnitine (LAC), 155, 156
L-carnitine (LC), 84, 155, 156, 175
Lenzi, A., 156, 157
Lepidium meyenii, 159
Lewis, R.W., 56
Lifestyle, 9, 24, 30, 35, 91
Lycopene, 34, 154, 156

M

Maca, 159, 160
MacLeod, J., 56
Male factor, 1, 5–7, 9, 15, 23, 26, 30, 31, 33, 41, 82, 90, 91, 111, 175, 179, 180
Male infertility
classification of, 5–9, 41–42, 44, 55, 84, 89, 90, 119, 123, 128, 130, 136
epidemiology of, 6, 41–42, 63, 79, 90–91, 99, 135, 179
prevalence of, 2–9, 42, 63, 71, 79, 106, 111, 125
Man, 13, 14, 23–25, 29–30, 71, 121, 125, 149, 181
Maretti, C., 89–95
Martini, A.C., 92
Matorras, R., 34
McLeod, 148
Mears, E.M., 107, 109
Menkeveld, 16
Misuraca, L., 41–52
Monoski, M.A., 49

N

Naz, R., 156
Nonobstructive azoospermia, 27, 28, 141
Nutritional supplements, 153

O

Obesity, 9, 46, 71, 81, 89–95, 138, 167
Obstruction, 8, 9, 14, 15, 41–43, 47, 48, 56, 69, 82, 105
Ochsendorf, F.R., 157
Oligoasthenoteratospermia, 27, 83
Oligozoospermia, 7, 15, 16, 28, 59, 67–69, 157
Oliva, A., 59
Omega-3, 91, 92, 154, 158
Omega-6, 154, 158

P

Paduch, D.A., 66
Palan, P., 156
Pare, A., 55
Pathogenesis, 56–57, 81–82, 94, 107, 153
Pauli, E.M., 92
Paulis, G., 63–72, 105–112
Pescatori, E.S., 23–31
Peterson, A.C., 125
Physical agents, 23–26, 28, 29, 31, 35, 37, 43, 46, 55, 57–59, 64, 66, 94, 95, 100, 120, 179, 181, 182, 1639
Piubello, G.D., 135–142

Polycystic ovary syndrome, 166, 174
Polyunsaturated fatty acids
 (PUFAs), 94, 154, 158
Premature ejaculation, 179, 181

R
Radiation therapy, 148–149
Raijmakers, M.T., 157
Reactive oxygen species, 17, 18, 28–29,
 36, 81, 107, 153
Richenberg, J., 126
Rolf, C., 154
Rybar, R., 92

S
Safarinejad, M.R., 92, 158, 159
Schlegel, P.N., 50
Selenium, 154, 157, 158
Seminal oxidative stress, 153, 154
Serter, S., 125
Sexual dysfunctions, 28, 179, 180, 182
Sigman, M., 156
Silber, S.J., 48
Sperm
 count, 15, 16, 28, 33–37, 41, 59, 60, 79,
  81, 84, 91–93, 107, 110, 125, 146–148,
  155–157, 159, 160, 165, 174, 175
 DNA fragmentation, 92, 111–112,
  155, 157
 function tests, 17–19, 59
 parameters, 26, 35, 36, 58, 79,
  92, 154–156, 158
Sperm analysis, 13–19, 26, 28, 33, 84
Stamey, T.A.S., 107, 109
Stephen, F., 122
Sterility, 69, 89, 148, 173
Surgery, 2, 8, 25, 27, 43, 46, 52, 58, 83,
 121–122, 127, 128, 131, 132, 149
Surgical error, 59

T
Tan, I.B., 126
Teratozoospermia, 7, 8, 173
Testicular cancer, 29, 69, 123, 125–132,
 145, 146, 149, 174

Testicular microlithiasis, 27, 125–126
Testicular torsion, 18, 44, 45, 83,
 123–124, 136
Testicular trauma, 9, 18, 83, 126–127, 136
Testis, 9, 18, 25, 26, 28, 29, 42, 51, 56,
 120–129, 131, 132, 136, 139, 141,
 142, 149, 166, 182
Therapy, 33, 44, 45, 47–52, 64–72, 84–85,
 94–95, 102, 106, 110, 121, 129,
 140–142, 148–149, 154, 156, 157,
 159, 173, 181
Therond, P., 154
Thonneau, P., 8
Toxic agents, 9, 14, 16, 44–46, 56, 93, 94,
 110, 166, 167
Tuderti, G., 41–52
Turchi, P., 1–2, 5–9

U
Unexplained infertility, 30, 31, 59, 91, 100
Unexplained male infertility
 (UMI), 99–102, 175

V
Varicocele, 7–9, 25–27, 30, 31, 44–47,
 55–60, 83, 111, 112, 125, 156, 175
Vermeulen, A., 56
Vitamin C, 34, 154, 155, 157, 159
Vitamin E, 154–155, 157, 159

W
Workup, 7, 24, 27, 29–31, 102
World Health Organization
 (WHO), 5, 13–16, 24, 26, 35,
 89, 90, 95

Y
Y microdeletions, 47, 82, 174
Young, S.S., 42, 158

Z
Zinc, 59, 80, 107, 154, 158–159, 166
Zorgnotti, A.W., 56

The manufacturer's authorised representative in the EU is Springer Nature Customer Service Centre GmbH, Europaplatz 3, 69115 Heidelberg, Germany. If you have any concerns regarding our products, please contact ProductSafety@springernature.com

Printed and bound by CPI Group (UK) Ltd, Croydon, CR0 4YY
23/03/2026
02076667-0012